Foreword to

It is only five years si⟶ ⟵d
on behalf of The Na⟶ ⟵n
has been fully updated and this has ⟶ ⟵e
revision of existing chapters. New sections have also been
added explaining more clearly the benefits and hazards of
obstetric intervention during labour; discussing the needs of
babies in Special Care and how to establish breastfeeding in
such circumstances; paying more attention to postnatal exercise
and to stress incontinence; and attempting to cover the topic of
pre-pregnancy care, in which increasing interest is being
shown by those women who come to The National Childbirth
Trust.

There seems every prospect that this second edition will
prove as popular, if not more so, than the first. Once again it
reminds us of the important role that The National Childbirth
Trust is playing in childbirth education in this country.

In spite of the relative abundance of baby books, *Pregnancy &
Parenthood* will be read with considerable interest by many
mothers, not only those who attend National Childbirth Trust
classes, since it represents the general view of The National
Childbirth Trust on so many vital topics concerned with
modern maternity care.

Norman Morris MD, FRCOG
Professor of Obstetrics and Gynaecology
Charing Cross Hospital Medical School

Contents

PREGNANCY

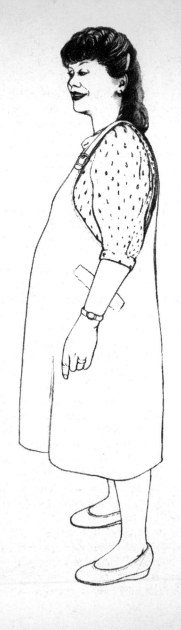

Introduction

Most women know little about pregnancy until they embark on it for the first time. If you have planned the pregnancy, you may well be more knowledgeable about contraception than about the conception and development of the fetus you are carrying. Some of the outward signs of early pregnancy, as they affect the mother, are well known—missed periods, morning sickness, and tiredness—but little emphasis is placed on the concurrent fascinating development of the unborn child, which is recognizably human from a very early stage and is remarkably complex. And however much you know in theory about pregnancy and parenthood, actually experiencing it is something new for each individual.

During the nine months of pregnancy the baby's bodily systems mature to the point where he can sustain life independent of the womb. Although at first you can be quite unaware of being pregnant, later you are constantly aware of the baby as he takes up more room in your body and his kicks and stretchings become stronger. Throughout pregnancy, the two of you are bound up together: the changes in his body directly cause changes in yours, and your health affects his development.

The culmination of pregnancy is giving birth, which is also a starting-point, or changeover point, as the expectation of parenthood becomes a reality. You will want to learn how to make this climax as rewarding as possible for yourself and as easy as possible for the baby. To do this you can learn relaxation and calm breathing patterns which will help your body to work more efficiently during labour and can act as a temporary distraction from the power of your labour should this be necessary to maintain your relaxation.

In order to check that everything is going well with the pregnancy, you should take full advantage of the comprehensive antenatal care available to all expectant mothers in this country. You and your baby both benefit from these check-ups, inconvenient though they may sometimes be. Be persistent in requesting sufficient information to answer all your questions.

Especially if this is your first pregnancy, you will find yourself reappraising your ideas about pregnancy, giving birth, and parenthood as the time for decision-making approaches and with it the realization that the responsibility is yours. You will find out for yourself that generalizations are just that: not everyone suffers from morning sickness or backache or food cravings; you do have some control over the amount of weight you put on; you can choose between the courses selected by your two friends, one of whom had an epidural, didn't feel a thing, and thought it was wonderful, the other who did without drugs and said that although it was hard work and hurt at times she certainly wouldn't have missed the marvellous sensations when her baby was actually born. You will find yourself reflecting on your own childhood: the times you thought your parents were perfect and the times you thought that if you ever had children you wouldn't expect them to do . . . All these decisions are now yours to make and it is important for your own sake not to let them go by default and later wish you had asked more questions or stuck to your own ideas.

Pregnancy affects the physical and emotional aspects of sexuality. The key to most problems of this nature is patience, linked with a willingness to explore new ways of lovemaking, and an understanding of what causes these temporary difficulties.

However much you have longed for a baby, there are always adjustments to be made when a couple is in the process of being transformed into a family. It is often hard for a woman to accept what she may regard as the 'inferior' role of motherhood, after the stimulus and responsibility of a full-time job. But the more you learn about it, the more you will come to realize how challenging and stimulating parenthood can be. You will also be in a position to make the best possible decisions for yourself and your baby.

This book is written for fathers as well as mothers. At last it has become respectable for men to take an active caring interest in their wives' pregnancies (though they have probably done so throughout history, albeit less openly than they do now), and for them to provide invaluable help and support when their children are born.

To those parents who have girl babies we offer apologies for the use of 'he' when referring to the baby. Our various attempts to move away from this all seemed at least intrusive and at worst confusing, so were abandoned.

Conception and development of the fetus

Your baby began as a single cell; when he is born, roughly 266 days later, this one cell will have multiplied to have become 200 million highly specialized cells in the complex body of a tiny human being.

In a sense, each new life has no definite beginning. Its existence is inherent in the existence of the parent cells and these, in turn, have arisen from the preceding parent cells. When any two parent cells unite, they bring together a blend of the attributes of all ancestors before them. Your baby is a completely new individual—not just a mixture of his parents' features but of characteristics which can be traced back through many generations. He is a link with the past and with the future.

The egg and the sperm

The female egg comes from the mother's ovary. She has two ovaries, each containing about a quarter of a million immature egg cells. Normally, one egg ripens each month in alternate ovaries, approximately two weeks before a menstrual period. The ripe egg bursts out of the ovary and falls into the trumpet-shaped opening of the Fallopian tube, which has an internal diameter the thickness of a cat's whisker and is about 10 cm

(4 in) long. One tube leads from each ovary to the thimble-sized cavity of the uterus, or womb. The minute round egg is slowly wafted towards the uterus by a gentle current of fluids within the tube. The egg has a very brief life and disintegrates unless it is fertilized and activated by a male cell on the first or second day after its arrival in the tube.

The male cells, or sperm, are produced in the father's testicles. At least 20 million and often as many as 500 million sperm cells may be present in a single ejaculation, but probably only a few dozen of the original millions released during

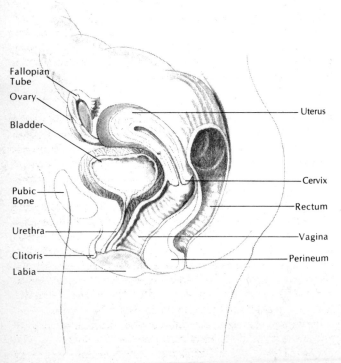

Fallopian Tube
Ovary
Bladder
Pubic Bone
Urethra
Clitoris
Labia

Uterus
Cervix
Rectum
Vagina
Perineum

The female reproductive organs

intercourse ever reach the egg, high up in the Fallopian tube. The male cells are much smaller than the egg and are often likened to miniature tadpoles because they look similar and can swim by lashing their tails backwards and forwards. It has been estimated that some male cells can travel the 17-cm (7-in) distance from the vagina to the Fallopian tubes in a little over an hour. A powerful enzyme helps one sperm to 'eat' its way through the outer membrane holding the substance of the egg, then through a finer underlying membrane holding the substance of the egg, until it reaches the centre and fuses with the maternal cell nucleus. Then a coating forms round the fertilized egg and prevents other sperm cells from entering.

In the nuclei of the sperm and the egg there are many thousands of genes which carry the 'instructions' or specifications for the design of every part of the new baby. With so many genes there can obviously be a virtually infinite number of variations on exisiting family patterns.

The first three months

By the end of the first week the original two cells which fused to form the fertilized egg have multiplied into a cluster of more than a hundred cells and have become implanted in the inner lining of the uterus. (If no egg is implanted in this lining, it disintegrates and is shed with the unfertilized egg during menstruation.)

By the end of the first month a complete, recognizable embryo has formed. It is only one centimetre ($\frac{1}{4}$–$\frac{1}{2}$ in) long but already has a head with rudimentary eyes, ears, mouth, and a brain. It has simple kidneys, a liver, a digestive tract, a primitive umbilical cord, the beginnings of a beating heart, and its own bloodstream. It is surrounded by an amnion or bag of waters, and is enclosed in a capsule covered with hundreds of root-like tufts which channel food from the lining of the uterus.

By the seventh week the embryo bears the familiar features and all the internal organs of the future adult, even though he is only 2 cm (less than an inch) long and weighs about a gramme ($\frac{1}{32}$ oz). He has a human face with eyes, ears, nose, lips, tongue,

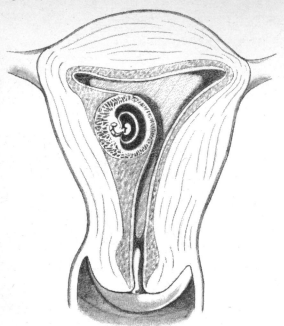

6-week embryo (actual size)

and even milk teeth buds in the gums. The body has become rounded, padded with muscles, and covered by a thin skin. The tiny arms have hands with fingers and thumbs, and the slower-growing legs have recognizable knees, ankles, and toes. The brain sends out impulses to co-ordinate the functioning of the other organs and the muscles of the arms and body can already be set in motion. The heart beats sturdily, the stomach produces digestive juices, the liver manufactures blood cells, and the kidneys extract uric acid from the blood.

During this period of teeming cell growth, the new cells are especially vulnerable to all physical and chemical influences, and diseases can be communicated from the mother. For this

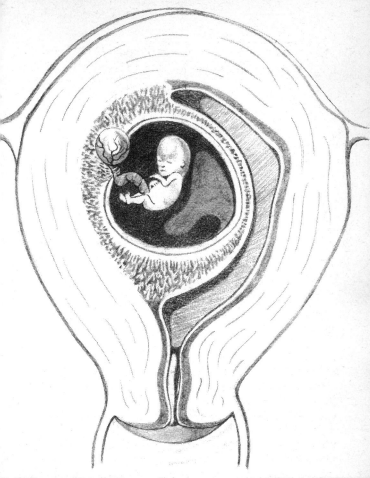

10-week embryo (actual size)

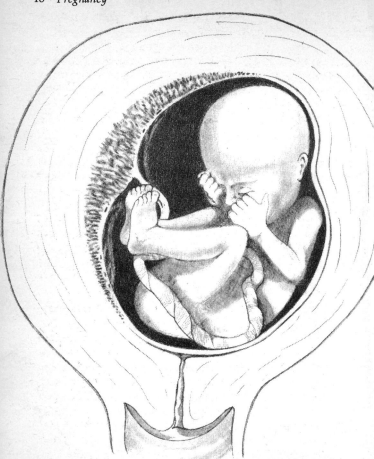

14-week baby in the uterus, showing placenta (actual size)

reason you should avoid exposure to known infectious diseases, take no drugs without medical advice, and avoid X-rays. It is wise to avoid these risks altogether as soon as you are planning to conceive, or think you have conceived, a child, even before you have missed a period. To some extent nature provides its own cure: if an embryo fails to grow properly, the 'mistake' is often rectified by an early miscarriage.

During the third month after conception, the baby begins to be quite active, although he is still so tiny that he would easily fit into a goose's egg and weighs only 28 g (1 oz). You are very unlikely to be able to feel your baby's movements because he is so small that the uterus has barely expanded and is still contained within the girdle of your hip-bones. However, by the end of the third month he can kick his legs, turn his feet, curl and fan his toes, make a fist, move his thumb, open his mouth, and press his lips tightly together. He will swallow considerable amounts of amniotic fluid and may even 'breathe' it in and out of his primitive lungs.

From the fourth to the sixth month

During the fourth to fifth month you will probably feel the baby turning and kicking against your sensitive abdominal wall. The uterus will have risen out of the confines of your pelvis and the baby will be much stronger. These first-perceived movements are called 'quickening' and can be a very exciting milestone in your pregnancy. In the fourth month the baby grows so much that he reaches half the height he will be at birth. He becomes 20–25 cm (8–10 in) tall but still weighs only about 170 g (6 oz). He is nourished through the umbilical cord which is attached to the placenta, which in turn is rooted in the lining of the uterus. The placenta is the organ through which the immature fetus receives oxygen and nutrients from your body, and also immunizing antibodies to combat infection, some of them produced by the placenta itself. The placenta is the main source of the hormones produced by your body in pregnancy which prepare for birth and the production of milk. Substances like alcohol, nicotine, and other drugs which enter your bloodstream may be transferred by the placenta to the baby within an hour or two.

In the fifth month the baby gains about 5 cm (2 in) in height and 28 g (10 oz) in weight. By the end of the month he will be about 30 cm (12 in) tall and will weigh about 500 g (1 lb). Fine downy hair starts to grow, the skeleton hardens, and the nails begin to form. His heartbeat may be heard if an ear is placed next to your abdominal wall: fathers and siblings can now also feel him kicking, turning, and jerking rhythmically with hiccups. The baby will now find a characteristic position in which he prefers to sleep, but he may be stirred into activity by loud external noises or vibrations.

In the sixth month he will become about 35 cm (14 in) tall and will start to accumulate fat under his skin. His weight will increase to about 800 g (1¾ lb). He can open and close his eyes and develops a strong grip with his hands. He has a chance of surviving in an incubator if born prematurely.

The last three months

In these months the baby gains most of his birthweight and outgrows his home in the uterus. He usually puts on about 500 g (1 lb) in the seventh month and nearly 2 kg (4½ lb) in the following six weeks. He develops a protective padding of fat which will help to keep his body warm after birth. He may begin to practise sucking (some babies are born with a callus on the thumb from sucking it *in utero*). He will probably settle into a head-down position and his body will fill the uterus. When he moves, the contours of his arms and legs can be felt and seen as bulges on your abdomen. During the last three months important immunizing agents to the diseases you have had or have been immunized against are transferred from you to the baby in the form of antibodies. These may be reinforced after birth by similar antibodies in your milk and its forerunner, colostrum. By the time these immunities wear off, at about six months of age, the baby's own system can cope better with infections and can begin to build up immunities of its own.

In the last month before birth, the expanded uterus sinks

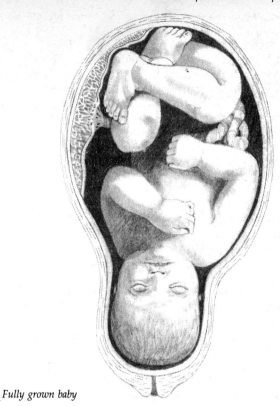

Fully grown baby

about 5 cm (2 in) downwards in your body and the baby's head (or buttocks) become engaged in the circle of your pelvic bones. This is called 'lightening' and will help to relieve the pressure of the baby underneath your rib-cage.

The baby's growth slows down as birth approaches—beauti-fully timed so that the baby becomes mature enough to be born just when he is still small enough to negotiate his exit.

Posture, muscle control, and general relaxation in pregnancy

As your figure changes and your baby grows, extra strain is put on some of your joints and muscles. This is due partly to the extra weight they must support and partly to a natural softening by the hormones which prepare your body for birth. A few simple exercises will help the muscles to become more supple but prevent them from becoming overstretched. Extra attention to the way you stand, sit, and move will prevent unnecessary strain, particularly on the joints of your back. During labour you will be able to relax your muscles and calm your breathing so that you can keep the rest of your body in harmony with the activities of your uterus.

Muscles and joints are not the only parts of your body that work harder during pregnancy; most of your internal organs are also more active. For example, your heart has to pump more blood round your body and your kidneys have to dispose of more waste matter. Most women are able to take these extra activities in their stride, but feel and look better if they live at a slightly slower pace and watch their diets with care.

Posture

Good posture changes and adjusts as movement of the limbs takes place. As you increase in size, your centre of gravity will change, therefore your posture will have to alter. The body is made with postural muscles and it is the maintenance of good posture which allows these muscles to remain strong and in good tone. At the end of the day your body will feel less tired if good posture has been maintained both in standing and sitting.

Lying If lying down causes breathlessness, dizziness, or bad heartburn, relief may be gained by lying on your side and being propped up from the waist, with pillows under your ribs, head, and shoulders. If the number of pillows under the head only is increased, a stiff neck may be added to your other problems! If

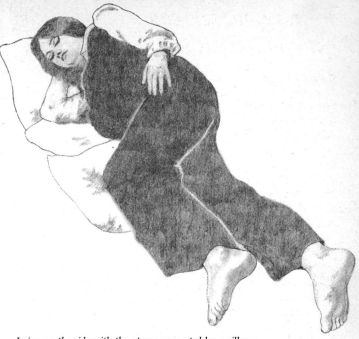

Lying on the side with the uterus supported by a pillow

your top hip aches, a small soft cushion may be put under the top knee, or under the bulge so that the uterus is supported in its correct position. On getting up, you should swing your legs over the side of the bed and sit on it for a few moments before you stand, so that you do not feel dizzy. After the first six or seven months of your pregnancy you should avoid lying flat on your back: it can affect your circulation and make you very faint. At the antenatal clinic do ask for pillows or for the head of the couch to be raised.

Kneeling Kneeling may be an extremely comfortable position from which to watch television or read, but it is important not to sit back on your heels unless there is a thick cushion on them, so

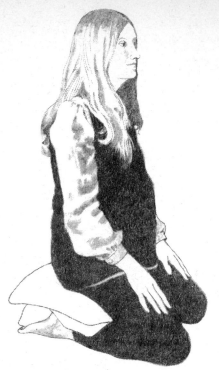

Kneeling with cushions behind the knees

that pressure behind the knees is avoided. Squatting with the knees apart is another potentially dangerous position because it is easy to overbalance; so if you wish to use this position, squat, sitting on a pile of cushions or a low stool. Some women find this very comfortable for relieving backache.

Sitting   The bones of the spine must be supported properly, either by their own muscles or by cushions. The most comfortable positions are probably either sitting on a hard chair at a table, with your elbows resting on the table to lift your rib-cage

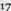

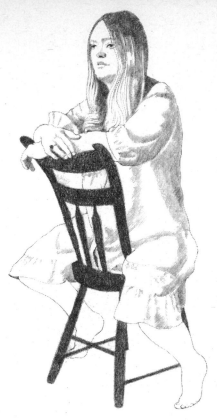

Comfortable sitting position in late pregnancy

and prevent excess pressure from the bulge on the lower ribs, or sitting on a narrow chair the wrong way round, your legs astride the seat, and your arms resting on the chair back. You could also try sitting on a low chair, such as a nursing chair, or on a soft, higher armchair with cushions behind your back, and your elbows supported on the chair arms. In a car, it is often most comfortable to sit on a cushion to prevent pressure in the groin area. When resting with the feet up, it is important to ensure that they are raised high enough—at least level with your bottom—and that there is no pressure in the groin. Support under your heels and knees (so that your knees are slightly bent) can be very comfortable.

Standing and walking Standing still should be avoided: the household chores should be done sitting or kneeling on a stool or the floor. When it is absolutely necessary to stand, keep the legs a little apart and take the body weight from one foot to the other; or, slowly rise up on your toes and come down again. There is always a tendency to compensate for the extra weight of your baby by leaning back, either from your ankles or from the waist. As your figure changes you will find it necessary to guard against these tendencies, particularly when you are tired. Make yourself as tall as you can, pull your abdomen in slightly and tuck your 'tail' down as in the pelvic rocking exercise described on p. 22, and make sure that your weight is evenly balanced between the balls and heels of your feet. This posture should be maintained while walking. When shopping it is a good idea to check your reflection in plate-glass windows to make sure you are standing correctly—what feels right may not always look right.

Lifting Stooping to lift a toddler, or a bag of shopping, can cause strain on the back. If you have a toddler, try to avoid lifting him, as far as possible. Teach him to climb safely in and out of his chair, and how to cope with the stairs. If he needs a cuddle, sit on a chair beside him, or kneel on the floor to bring yourself down to his level. If you want to pick up something from the floor, crouch, keeping your knees together, or kneel on one knee; pick up the object and then use your thigh muscles to straighten you up, pushing off with your hand on the floor or on your knee. If you have to carry a lot of shopping, always use two bags, one in each hand, to balance the weight, and when you pick them up, bend your knees or kneel on one knee, and use your legs to straighten up, not your back muscles.

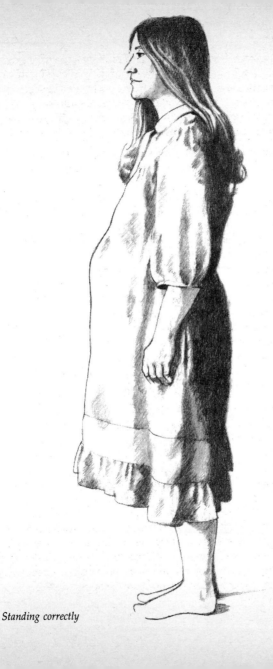

Standing correctly

With the approval of your doctor or midwife exercises can be started after you are 16 weeks pregnant. It should only be necessary to spend about 10–15 minutes each day on the exercises, as several of the movements should become part of your daily lifestyle. Practise each exercise six times, counting four slowly as you do each movement and four as you return to your starting position. Provided there is no discomfort, always contract and relax each group of muscles as much as you can each time. *If you have any pain, bleeding, or illness, stop practising all the exercises until you have been medically examined.*

To prevent overstretching of the abdominal wall

Lie back, pillows under your head and shoulders, with your knees bent and feet flat. Tighten your abdominal muscles so that the baby is pulled gently down towards your backbone. Relax slowly. Try to make a habit of tightening and relaxing your abdominal muscles in this way at intervals during the day when you are standing and sitting, particularly if you notice a 'sagging' feeling. If practised regularly this exercise is a great help towards getting your figure back after your baby is born.

To teach awareness (control) of the pelvic floor

A woman normally uses pelvic floor muscles around and deep inside the vagina during intercourse—often without being really aware of what she is doing. Increasing awareness of the actions of these muscles encourages relaxation during delivery and quick recovery of muscle tone afterwards. The following exercise will help you to locate and feel the muscles moving. Get into the same position as for the previous exercise, or sit on a low chair, leaning forward with your arms resting on your knees. Tighten the ring of muscles around your anus (back passage) as though you were trying to stop yourself passing a motion; make sure that your abdominal and buttock muscles remain relaxed. Let go. Now, tense then relax the muscles which surround the urethra and vagina (front passage and birth canal). You may recognize this as a muscle movement you make during intercourse. You use the same muscles when you need to pass water and are trying to hold on. A good test of their strength therefore is to try to 'stop the stream' for a moment when urinating. Now contract both sets of muscles together, thus pulling up the whole of the pelvic floor (the sling of muscle which surrounds the passages and supports your pelvic organs). Relax slowly and completely and then lift these muscles back to their normal position. Make this exercise another of your regular habits, particularly if you have to stand for some time and notice a heaviness between your legs.

Preparing for the birth of your baby's head

(a) Rest on your bed with your knees bent, your feet and knees wide apart, and your back supported by several pillows. Gradually relax your thighs and pelvic floor muscles so that your knees fall more and more widely apart (your feet will roll gently on to their outer borders). Leave your legs in this position. At first it may seem unnatural and uncomfortable, but after a little practice you will get the correct feeling of 'letting go' and can practise panting, as you will be asked to do when it is time for your baby's head to pass slowly and gently out of the birth canal. You can practise this also in a kneeling position (see p. 57) and a 'supported squatting' position (see p. 56).

(b) Position yourself as for (a) but with your feet and knees together. Press your knees together hard and, at the same time, tighten the pelvic floor muscles as in the first exercise. Note the feeling of tension along the inner sides of your thighs and between your legs; many women tense involuntarily when their babies' heads are stretching the outlet of the birth canal. Relax, and notice carefully the different feel of the muscles; this is the feeling to aim for when you are giving birth.

(c) 'Squatting' on a low stool (see illustration on p. 65). Let yourself relax in this position. It can be very comfortable in pregnancy as well as being a preparation for the second stage of labour.

To relieve backache

Sit on the front of a firm chair, leaning on your hands at the back

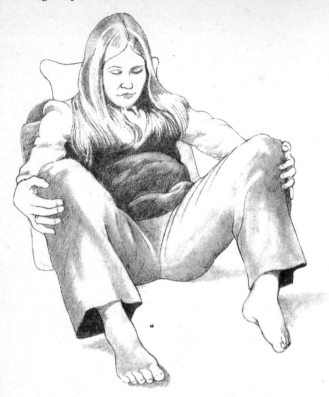

Exercise position to prepare for the birth of the baby's head

of the seat. Hollow your back slightly; notice how your pelvis tilts down in front. Now round your back as much as you can; notice how your pelvis tilts up in front and your 'tail' is pulled well down at the back. Try the exercise standing up and lying down.

If you have backache, particularly the kind where you get 'locked' if you sit or lie for a long time, try 'unlocking' yourself

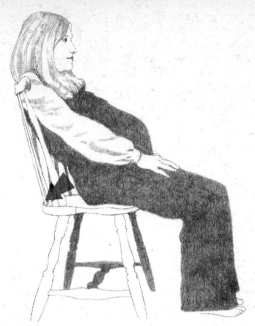

Pelvic rocking while seated on a chair

by doing this pelvic rocking movement a few times before you attempt to change your position. If you suffer from backache during labour, try sitting on your side and do the rocking very, very gently, in time with your breathing; or better still, kneel, leaning on the seat of a chair, or the bed trolley, and rock in this position.

Relaxation

Muscle tension can be an appropriate and necessary response in times of emergency. Tension allowed to become a way of life is, however, counter-productive. It consumes energy you might put to better use; it can lead to dependence on alcohol, cigarettes, or tranquillizers. During pregnancy in particular you will want to avoid these hazards and conserve your energy: pregnancy brings with it its own physical and emotional demands. An ability acquired now, to recognize your own responses to stress and overcome them, will be of use to you in the long term too.

Are you aware of your own responses to stress? Do you tense your shoulders, clench your teeth or fists, get a tight feeling in your throat, become unjustifiably ill-tempered, sigh frequently, curl up your toes? If you have been in the habit of smoking or drinking you may well be deficient in vitamins B and C: see diet section.

The aim of the following suggestions is to help you to

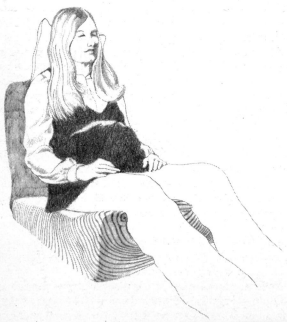

Position for practising relaxation, showing NCT 'wedge'

recognize the difference between tension and relaxation: the tightness of a muscle which is working compared with the feeling you have when it is at rest. It is not difficult to learn this and once you have mastered it you can put it into practice wherever you are whenever you become aware of your own tension (for example even sitting in a traffic jam).

For practice sessions, ideally use a comfortable chair, with a high back to support your head, so that you can rest or sleep afterwards. Do not try to hurry—that would defeat the objective.

Some ways to practise relaxation

1. Sit well back in a chair, with your feet flat on the floor or your legs and feet supported on a stool. Close your eyes. Stretch your heels away from you—legs as long and straight as you can make them. Stop doing this. Wriggle your toes, and then rock your legs from side to side. Let your feet and legs rest still.

2. Stretch your hands away from you—fingers, hands, and arms stretched, with your shoulders coming forwards as well. Let your hands rest on your lap again. Wriggle your fingers, then raise your hands and shake them as though you are flicking drops of water from your fingers. Let your hands and arms rest again.

3. As briskly as you can, mouth (silently) the numbers from one to ten—do it again. Repeat, mouthing the numbers very slowly: notice the strong movements of your lips. Then frown, grit your teeth together, and screw your eyes tight shut. Follow this by raising your eyebrows and stretching your mouth wide. Relax again and then let your head roll gently from side to side a few times.

4. Push your bottom and back hard into the chair which is supporting you, and then stop so that your body rests comfortably and your muscles are relaxed.

5. Tighten the muscles of your pelvic floor—the muscles surrounding the anus, vagina, and urethra. Hold them tight for a few seconds and then let them go back to their normal position.

With all these five points you will probably notice that as you tighten your muscles you automatically hold your breath, and as you relax you breathe out. This shows you how closely related breathing and relaxation are. Try to remember the feeling you get from a tense muscle and the very different feeling you get from a relaxed muscle. Soon you will be able to recognize tension instantly. Practise keeping your breathing regular as well. Calm breathing promotes the release of unnecessary muscle tension.

Whilst the contrast between muscle tightening, or stretching, and relaxation is useful as a learning technique, repeated tightening of the muscles can, for some people, result in increased tension instead of relaxation, so aim to do without it. Enlist the help of a partner if possible and practise together.

6. To continue with your relaxing, massage may help you. With both hands stroke gently across your face, from your neck up over your lower jaw, up over your cheeks, and out to the corners of your eyes; repeat this several times. Then smooth your fingertips across your forehead and out to your temples; repeat this several times. Then let your hands rest on your lap. Remember the feeling of warmth and smoothness.

7. In the same way, sense a deep peace and calm spreading from the base of your spine, up your back, and out to the point of your shoulders. Let it continue down your arms and into your hands and feel your hands and fingers becoming warmer.

With a partner you could try doing massage in these places: over the face, and in a big sweeping movement up the back and down the arms; or using alternate hands in a continuous rhythm down the back from shoulders to buttocks. You would need to find a comfortable position to lie in, or sit leaning forwards so that your partner could reach your back easily. Try it both ways; you massaging your partner and then your partner massaging you. If you are massaging bare skin, some hand cream or oil will help your hands to slide smoothly over it.

8. If possible have a rest once you have practised these techniques—perhaps even a sleep. Before opening your eyes, think about how you feel now and enjoy the feeling of being

relaxed. Move gently, stretching, wriggling your fingers and toes, yawning if you need to. Slowly open your eyes and continue to enjoy your relaxed feelings as you become aware of your surroundings and responsibilities again.

At night you may like to practise relaxing before you go to sleep. If sleep remains evasive—try to become aware of your own breathing: of the breaths coming into and going out of your body, as you let go a little more with each one . . . If your mind is very active then try to concentrate on a pleasant picture which involves a simple movement of your eyes—for example a long pendulum swinging slowly from side to side; or a ball bouncing very high, slowly—something you find soothing. Listening to music might help, or having a warm bath, a small snack, or a warm drink.

Problems of pregnancy

The major physical characteristic of pregnancy is the swelling of your abdomen into what most mothers call their 'bulge' or 'bump'. However, other complex bodily changes are taking place which are not so obvious. Both the sheer size of the growing 'bump' and these other changes can cause discomforts, most of which can be alleviated in some way.

Care of your body

Relaxin, the relaxing hormone which is produced during pregnancy, affects all body structures. It loosens joints, so take care not to strain them. Activities such as walking, swimming, and dancing are very good but a programme of strenuous exercises is not advisable, particularly if you are not used to them. It is very important to check your posture: that in itself is good exercise for your muscles.

The hormone also slows down the digestive and excretory systems, so eat smaller, more frequent meals and drink plenty of water, which helps to prevent constipation. Roughage is important—added bran in cereals and home baking, plus raw fruits and vegetables, help to prevent constipation. Eat at least one raw meal every day, such as a fruit or vegetable salad, and if constipation persists try taking a mixture of dried fruits and senna powder.

Relaxin slows the return circulation and can produce *varicose veins*. You can help to prevent these by doing some simple exercises anytime, anywhere:

Draw circles with your toes, moving from the ankle—right foot goes clockwise, left foot anticlockwise—thereby strengthening the muscles which support the long arch of your foot;

Make gripping movements with your toes: you can even do this standing with your shoes on;

Sitting or lying: point your toes downwards, hard, then turn them up towards your knees;

If necessary ask your doctor for a prescription for support hose—there are some which can be made to measure so that the length is correct for you. Wearing a lightweight pantie girdle during the last six to eight weeks of pregnancy supports the baby's weight when it has a considerable weight gain; it also helps to prevent overstretching of the abdomen and strain on the lower back, both of which tend to cause bad posture, and the resulting pressure makes varicose veins worse. (Vitamin E capsules can help to get rid of varicose veins. Ask your doctor about them.) If wearing a girdle seems a nuisance or bothers you, wear one when you are busy, and remove it when you are resting.

The rib-cage enlarges by 8–10 cm (3–4 in) round its lower part towards the end of pregnancy and can cause *backache, shoulder*, and *rib pain*. To avoid this, your back should be straight——whether sitting, lying, standing, or kneeling.

Be careful about your posture when doing housework. Try sitting or kneeling on a stool at the sink instead of standing, sitting to prepare vegetables, kneeling to make the bed, and bending your knees rather than your back when you pick up objects from the floor. Try cleaning the bath when you are in it, instead of hanging over the side to do it.

Stretching both arms above your head for any length of time, lying flat on your back, having hot baths, and getting up too quickly from a lying or sitting position, can cause fainting. Sitting slumped in a chair may cause backache and indigestion, standing for too long increases the likelihood of varicose veins, and squatting right down on your heels with the legs apart exerts great pressure on the muscles at the base of the pelvis and may cause you to overbalance.

Dry, flaking, itching skin can be relieved by massaging in body lotion, almond oil, or other creams. When trying one you have not used before, put it on only a very small area of skin first in case it causes a rash. *Itching* may be relieved by using a lotion made by steeping nettle leaves in hot water and then letting the liquid cool before applying it (see also p. 31). *Stretch marks* on the sides of the breasts may be avoided if you wear a sleep bra at night.

Minor ailments in pregnancy

catarrh	try a weak inhalation, garlic perles or sugar-coated garlic tablets, biochemic tissue salts (Combination Q).
bleeding gums	try massaging them with your fingertips before brushing with a soft bristle brush.
indigestion	try eating smaller meals, sitting up very straight to eat them, and taking heartburn mixture (which works faster than tablets) *obtained on prescription from your doctor.*
backache	try correcting your posture, and wearing a light-weight girdle to support the weight of the baby, which eases sciatic and other similar pains. Try kneeling on all fours, or with your arms on the seat of a

chair, and wag your tail from side to side. Use a kidney-shaped plastic box of the type made to help children stand at a wash-basin and sit or kneel-sit, rocking your pelvis forwards and backwards.

piles

first cure any constipation (see pp. 27–8); don't strain. Try a suppository of peeled garlic, retained overnight. Vitamin E may help.

swollen ankles

don't stand still; try sitting on a high chair, or on a cushion when in the car, so that there is less pressure in your groin. Whenever you sit down put your feet up—legs comfortably supported.

cramp

stretch the affected part, then quickly bend it; to avoid further attacks don't drink milk at bedtime, and stretch as you wake up with your heels down and toes up. Hip cramp may be relieved by taking your weight equally on both feet, especially when rising from a sitting position—say, from a chair or a car seat.

weight gain

with a correctly balanced diet and plenty of raw fruit and vegetables, wholewheat bread, and wholegrain cereals, weight gain should be normal: currently the recommendation is a gain of approximately 12.5–16 kg (28–35 lb).

stretch marks

cannot be prevented but may be kept to a minimum by keeping the skin

supple (using cream or oil),
correcting posture, and having
adequate support for the abdomen
and breasts. Vitamin E oil may help
remove scars when rubbed into
them.

varicose veins
avoid standing still, wearing tight
garments, and being constipated. Try
a high-fibre diet and a vitamin E
supplement.

aching feet
do foot exercises (circling the feet,
pointing the toes, drawing up the
toes), and avoid standing still for
long. 'Exercise' sandals can damage
your feet and can make you trip
up—avoid them.

feeling faint
avoid moving too quickly from a
lying or sitting position, avoid smoky
atmospheres and long journeys, and
increase the iron intake in your diet.

itching (like thrush,
see p. 29 for other
itching)
may be relieved by applying natural
yoghurt to the vaginal area.

nausea/'morning
sickness'
can occur at any time of day. See
'Diet in pregnancy' section for
guidelines to alleviate it. Some
doctors think taking iron tablets can
cause sickness.

fatigue
may occur in early and late
pregnancy and it is important not to
force yourself to do too much. If you
cannot have a daily rest lying down,
alternate periods of activity with
periods of rest, and do not plan any

appointments, especially evening appointments, which you cannot cancel.

abdominal or round ligament pain

pain below the 'bump', in the groin, is due to ligament strain and may be alleviated by wearing a lightweight pantie-girdle or properly designed maternity support (ask about this at your antenatal clinic); resting with the feet up, with a pillow under the hips and under the head and shoulders; and taking great care over walking downstairs and downhill (especially if holding a push-chair or shopping trolley).

pelvic discomfort

again, a lightweight girdle and correct posture will help, as will frequently repeated pelvic floor exercises (see p. 20).

vaginal discharge

is increased during pregnancy (usually white), but any offensive green, yellow, or bloodstained discharge should be reported to your doctor.

insomnia

having a small snack at bedtime, a warm bath, a hot water bottle, plenty of supporting pillows (see pp. 14–15), and cat-napping, assisted by relaxation and comfortably deep breathing, may all help.

contact lenses

it may be necessary to discontinue the use of these during pregnancy. If in doubt, consult your optician.

bladder discomfort

the baby may appear to be rubbing

his head on your bladder, causing
soreness. 'Kneel-sitting' (see p. 15)
on a pillow on your heels may
relieve it, or sitting on a low stool.

See also homoeopathy section (p. 286).

Antenatal medical procedures

Whether you wish to have your baby at home or in hospital the
pattern of antenatal medical care should be similar. Report to
your doctor as soon as you think that you may be pregnant so
that you can confirm the diagnosis and start planning for the
birth of your baby. The sooner you do this, the better for your
health and the baby's.

The first antenatal examination

During your first antenatal consultation the doctor or midwife
will ask you questions about the details of any previous
pregnancies, including miscarriages, abortions, previous
births, and ectopic (tubal) pregnancies, also twins in parents'
families or any abnormal babies; your general state of health;
how you feel now; past illnesses and operations; the medical
history of your immediate family; any medicines or drugs that
you may be taking; the date of your last menstrual period;
details of your usual menstrual cycle, and what kind of contraception you may have been using until the time that you
conceived.

The doctor will make a general physical examination: testing
your urine, noting your weight, height, blood pressure and the
state of your heart, lungs, breasts, and abdomen. If you have
reached the third month (12 weeks) of your pregnancy, the
doctor should be able to feel the top of your uterus just above
the pubic bone at the front of your pelvis. If your pregnancy is
less far advanced, enlargement, softening, and the change in

the shape of your uterus characteristic of pregnancy can only be detected by feeling the uterus with two hands (bi-manual examination). This is done with one hand feeling through your abdominal wall and with one or two fingers of the other hand feeling the cervix and lower part of your uterus through the vagina. Such a bi-manual pelvic or vaginal examination also

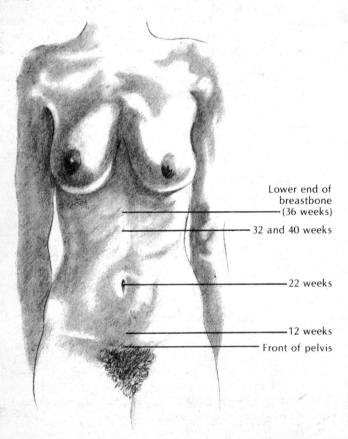

Lower end of breastbone (36 weeks)

32 and 40 weeks

22 weeks

12 weeks

Front of pelvis

Approximate height of uterus at different stages during pregnancy

gives the doctor some idea of the shape and size of your pelvis, whether or not you have any fibroids (common benign non-cancerous tumours of the uterine muscle)or cysts on the ovaries that may cause problems, as well as confirming the diagnosis and duration of the pregnancy. At this time the doctor may also use a speculum (a metal instrument) to look into the vagina and see the cervix. This gives the doctor an opportunity to take a cytological smear from the cervix for the detection of any early pre-cancerous changes, and also to detect any infections such as 'thrush' (candida or monilia) or TV (*Trichomonas vaginitis*), which cause an irritating unpleasant-smelling discharge.

If the doctor cannot be sure that you are pregnant, it is simple to carry out a pregnancy test on your urine. In special circumstances, it is also possible to have a very sensitive pregnancy test done on your blood. If you are pregnant, this test will show positive within ten days of conception, whereas pregnancy tests on urine are unlikely to give a positive result until 14 days after you have missed a period.

A vaginal examination carried out gently in early pregnancy does not provoke miscarriage, but if you are worried about this tell your doctor before he makes the examination. Having completed the examination, the doctor should tell you his findings and give you his opinion as to how the pregnancy can be expected to proceed. Now is the time to discuss with the doctor where you will have your baby and who will look after you during pregnancy and labour (see 'The choice of birth at home', p. 99).

However you are to be cared for, you may be given a Maternity Co-operation Card. You should carry this card with you not only when attending your antenatal clinic, but at all times during pregnancy in case you have an accident. It contains a summary of your medical history, any tests carried out, and the progress of your pregnancy, so that the midwife or doctor who sees you has all the relevant information, and can then make his or her own notes.

Blood tests

At the time of your first antenatal examination, or soon afterwards, blood tests are carried out to identify your blood group; to determine whether or not your blood contains any antibodies (for example, the Rhesus negative factor) that could affect the baby; to assess the haemoglobin level and detect anaemia; to exclude syphilis; to find out whether you are susceptible or resistant (immune) to German measles (rubella); and, if you come from Africa, Asia, or a Mediterranean country, to check whether your blood has any unusual haemoglobin (sickle cell test) which makes the red blood cells more fragile and causes anaemia.

Blood tests to estimate haemoglobin levels and detect any antibody formation are usually repeated later in pregnancy at 28 weeks and again at 36 weeks.

Blood tests may also be performed in early pregnancy to check alpha-feto-protein levels—see p. 40, 'Neural tube defects'.

Antenatal visits throughout pregnancy

During a normal pregnancy the doctor or midwife will ask to see you every four weeks from the first visit until 28 weeks, every two weeks from 28 weeks to 36 weeks, and then every week until the baby is born. If any abnormality is detected, or if you need special care, you may be asked to attend the antenatal clinic more frequently than this.

At each visit you will be asked how you feel. You will be weighed and have your blood pressure taken and your urine will be checked to make sure that there are no signs of problems. Your abdomen will be examined to see how the uterus is growing and later on how the baby is lying. If you are expecting a first baby, you will usually feel the baby move for the first time between 18 and 22 weeks. If you have had a baby before, you may feel it move for the first time as early as 16 weeks. Note the date and tell the doctor. The baby's heart can usually be heard with an ordinary fetal stethoscope at about 24 weeks. It can be heard much earlier than this, even before you are able to feel the baby's movements, if ultrasound is used to detect the beating heart.

Tests of fetal health and placental function

In a normal pregnancy with a healthy baby this is most easily measured by the steady increase in your weight, the quality and strength of the baby's movements, and the growth rate of your uterus. In some women the rate of growth of the pregnancy, and/or complicating medical conditions (such as high blood pressure, diabetes, previous stillbirths, premature deliveries, and trouble with a previous baby after birth) may cause concern. In such circumstances it may be desirable to follow the baby's progress as closely as possible to decide whether or not early delivery, perhaps by Caesarean section, might be in the baby's best interests. This can be done by fortnightly ultrasound measurement of the baby's head; repeated tests on your blood to measure the level of hormones such as oestrogen and HPL (human placental lactogen); repeated measurements in 24-hour collections of urine of the amount of oestrogens; recording the baby's heart-rate to see whether or not the pattern of activity and variation is normal, which is a guide to the state of the oxygen supply to the baby.

Estimation of pelvic shape and size

One of the aims of antenatal care is to detect any hindrance which might arise if the baby should be too big to pass through the pelvic bones and the birth canal. This is called cephalo-pelvic disproportion (disproportion of baby's head to mother's pelvis). In a healthy woman of normal height this is most unlikely; however, in women who are shorter than average the pelvic bones may be too small, and this may cause delay and difficulty in labour. In women expecting a first baby, the head usually settles into the pelvic cavity (engages) some time after 36 weeks and before labour begins. In a woman who has had one or more babies before, engagement of the head may not occur until labour starts. Her previous experience will be a guide to the width of her pelvis.

Many doctors do another routine pelvic examination during the last four weeks of pregnancy to make a clinical estimate of the shape and size of your pelvis in relation to the size of the baby's head. In a few women it may be necessary to find out much more about the pelvic shape and size from an X-ray. This may be suggested if you are very small, if the baby is thought to be very large, if the baby's head does not engage easily, or if you expect a breech delivery (see p. 133). Usually only one film is taken with you standing sideways on to the X-ray film with a ruler between your legs, so that the size of the pelvic outlet, cavity, and inlet can be measured directly from the film.

Ultrasonic examination

Using a source of very high frequency sound that cannot be heard by the human ear (ultrasound), it is possible to examine the contents of the uterus in pregnancy by plotting on a television screen how the ultrasound signals are reflected back from various surfaces such as the wall of the uterus, the placenta, the baby, and his beating heart. By measuring the size of the baby's head the duration of pregnancy can be estimated. If these measurements are repeated, the growth rate of the baby can be followed. The measurements usually made are of the baby's head size between the two bony prominences above the ears. Using ultrasound, the movements of the baby's heart can be detected before they can be heard, the situation of the placenta can be located, and if twins are present they can be detected. Neural tube defects such as spina bifida can also be seen. Some obstetricians ask every woman to have three ultrasound scans to measure the baby's growth rate so that the duration of pregnancy can be known as accurately as possible. Other obstetricians are more selective and only use ultrasound scans to obtain further information for special reasons, such as before amniocentesis; if more than one baby is suspected; if fetal death is suspected; if the growth rate of the baby is either too fast or too slow; if the menstrual dates are doubtful and there is a need to estimate the expected date of delivery more accurately; or if there has been bleeding and it is necessary to know whether the placenta is attached low down in the uterus (placenta praevia).

There is no evidence as yet that exposure of babies to ultrasound is harmful, but on the other hand there is no absolute proof that it is harmless. Those using ultrasound can misinterpret what is seen. Therefore some consultants believe that ultrasound is best used selectively for particular reasons, and that the scans should not be used as the only basis on which to make decisions.

Detection of congenital abnormalities before birth

About one in forty babies born alive has some physical defect. Most are minor, such as birthmarks, but some are serious, and a few do not allow the baby to survive or lead a normal independent life. Not all abnormalities can be detected before birth, particularly those of the heart and major blood vessels, and those of the limbs and digestive system.

If it is suspected that your baby may be at risk, special tests can be carried out to confirm or refute the possibility. Most of these tests involve a maternal alpha-feto-protein test first, followed, if necessary, by a procedure called amniocentesis (see below).

At present, if an abnormal baby is detected in pregnancy, nothing can be done to correct the physical deformities, although some organic and physiological conditions can be treated. The aim of detecting abnormal pregnancies is, therefore, to offer those concerned the opportunity of considering whether to continue with the pregnancy, or to have it terminated. If this is not a choice you would wish to consider, there is no point in having the tests carried out.

Amniocentesis This is the method used to obtain a sample of the amniotic fluid surrounding the baby. A local anaesthetic solution is injected to numb a small part of the mother's abdominal wall just below the umbilicus (navel). A needle is pushed through the numb part into the uterus taking care to avoid the placenta (which is first located by ultrasound) so that a small sample of the baby's amniotic fluid can be sucked out with a syringe for examination in the laboratory. Unfortunately this test is not without danger to the baby: one baby in a hundred is spontaneously aborted as a result of the test and a further one in seventy is damaged by it but survives. The test is also not completely reliable: it has been estimated that in 20 per cent of cases where the baby has a neural tube defect the level of alpha-feto-protein is not raised. Remember that even up to the age of forty there is only a one in a hundred chance of having an abnormal baby.

Neural tube defects   The commonest of the more serious defects (one in 200 births) involves the development of the spinal cord, spinal column, the brain, and the skull—so-called neural tube defects, which include spina bifida and anencephaly. Neural tube defects can be detected by testing the mother's blood between 16 and 22 weeks of pregnancy for alpha-feto-protein. If this is present in larger amounts than usual, it merely suggests that the baby may have a neural tube defect, but it is not conclusive evidence that this is so unless alpha-feto-protein is also found in abnormal quantities in the water (amniotic fluid) surrounding the baby. The alpha-feto-protein level of the mother's blood is also raised with a normal twin pregnancy or if the baby has died; it also rises as pregnancy progresses. Therefore, no attempt is usually made to obtain amniotic fluid for testing until the duration of the pregnancy has been checked and the possibility of twins has been excluded. This can most easily be done by ultrasound examination (see above), when the situation of the placenta (afterbirth) can also be located.

Down's syndrome (mongolism)   This is another abnormality that can be detected in pregnancy before the baby is born. Down's syndrome is caused by an abnormality in the baby's chromosomes, which store the genes, or blueprints for the structure and function of our cells. To detect or exclude Down's syndrome, the chromosome constitution of the baby is ascertained before it is born. Fluid obtained by amniocentesis will contain living cells shed from the baby's skin which can be isolated in the laboratory and grown in tissue culture. About three to four weeks later, when the cells divide, the chromosome pattern can be recognized. The tests required naturally cause anxiety, because they cannot be completed quickly and it is not usually possible to obtain water from around the baby by amniocentesis before 16 weeks. This means you will not know the answer until about 20 to 22 weeks of pregnancy. The abnormal chromosomes of Down's syndrome may be passed on to the baby if either parent is carrying this defect, or more commonly if the ovum (egg) is abnormal before it is fertilized, which is more likely to happen in women who become pregnant in later life.

Other abnormalities A few other rare abnormalities can be detected by tests on the amniotic fluid (for example Thalassaemia, an inherited abnormal haemoglobin causing anaemia). Tests on amniotic fluid can also be made on Rhesus negative women with antibodies to find out the best time for delivery, and whether or not the baby needs a transfusion in the uterus before birth. Amniotic fluid obtained by amniocentesis in late pregnancy (after 28 weeks) is also used to determine the maturity of the baby, particularly of his lungs, to know—if premature delivery is indicated—how well the baby is likely to be able to expand his lungs and breathe on his own.

Transcervical aspiration This is being used as a test for fetal abnormality which can be done earlier in pregnancy than amniocentesis. Some of the cells from the chorionic villi from which the placenta develops are removed and cultured to show up chromosomal abnormalities and some hereditary blood disorders as early as 6 to 8 weeks after conception. Because this is done so early in pregnancy more abnormal fetuses will be found, because those which would otherwise abort spontaneously will not have done so this early.

Ask for explanations

Throughout your pregnancy you are entitled to know, and you

should know, what is happening, why tests are necessary, and what the results are. At no time in pregnancy should anything be done to you unless you have received a full explanation which you have understood and willingly accepted. If you do not understand, ask for an explanation. If you are afraid of the tests in any way, say so. If you are not given an explanation that satisfies you, go on asking questions until you are satisfied. If necessary, enlist the aid of your partner. Antenatal care, unfortunately, easily becomes a mechanical and impersonal process for many doctors and midwives, unless you are prepared to question them and make it necessary for them to treat you as an individual. Make them aware tactfully that it is your baby, and that your fears and doubts may be as important as the results of any tests that are carried out.

Diet during pregnancy

It is not usually necessary to change your eating habits completely because you are pregnant, but most mothers take a new look at their diet and find that they can improve it one way or another. For any healthy person the basic aim is to eat a balanced, nutritious diet, as varied as you can make it. Eat sensibly from the different food groups daily; fresh fruit and vegetables, some wholegrain carbohydrates, proteins, and a little fat. Avoid eating too much of any one food or group or supplement. Improvements made to diet during pregnancy help to make the woman ready for motherhood—by preparing her for breastfeeding her baby and by giving her the physical and nervous energy necessary to look after him/her.

Advice for a wholesome diet

1. Avoid sugar and artificial additives, colouring and flavouring found in abundance in 'convenience' ready prepared foods, processed breakfast cereals, and bottled drinks and squashes.

Preservatives are used in many processed meats (bacon, sausages, Continental meats), so these are best avoided.

2. Many trace elements have been found essential for health and especially for the normal development of the baby. If you eat plenty of raw and unprocessed foods these will automatically be included in your diet.

3. Wholegrain flour and cereals and brown rice and pasta are more nutritious than refined products (although if you are accustomed to eating large amounts of white 'factory' bread you may need to make a gradual change to wholewheat as the chemicals may have produced a form of addiction and too rapid a change may cause digestive problems).

4. Fresh fruit and vegetables are higher in food values and are generally lower in cost than processed ones. Fruits and most vegetables are more nutritious eaten raw. Vitamin C is destroyed by heat and by prolonged exposure to the air once the skin is cut. To cook vegetables, steam or boil as briefly as possible in very little water to avoid loss of vitamins and minerals. Green leafy vegetables, for instance, should be shredded and cooked for not longer than three minutes to avoid loss of vitamins. Try to avoid using aluminium pans or teapots.

5. Limit fat and 'rich' meals, i.e. refined foods high in fat and sugar content, especially fried foods.

6. Allergens: if you are allergic to, or simply do not like, any particular foods then omit them from your diet—it is nourishment not the foodstuff which is necessary. Cow's milk and cheese, eggs, wheat, oranges, and tomatoes are common allergens and it may be necessary to choose sources of nourishment other than these, from the same food groups. If you eat a good mixed diet, then all foods will be taken in moderation. Foods taken in their natural state are a better source of nourishment and can be absorbed by the body because the balance is as nature intended. Avoid, as far as possible, food in cans, jars, and packets. Fruit (to be eaten unpeeled especially) needs to be well scrubbed under running water to remove the sprays which may have been used.

During pregnancy

Given a healthy well-balanced diet, what changes should a woman make when she becomes pregnant?

1. Calcium intake should be increased. Calcium is necessary for the development of the teeth and bones of the fetus. Teeth begin to form at 4–6 weeks of intra-uterine life, before you even know you are pregnant. The absorption of calcium by the fetus is mainly greater during the last three months, particularly the last 6–8 weeks of pregnancy, both from the maternal blood, through the placenta, and by drinking the amniotic fluid. Sources of calcium are given below.

2. Iron intake should be increased and needs extra vitamin C to help absorption. The B vitamins can be helpful in preventing constipation and skin problems. There is evidence that vitamin E may have some beneficial effects on blood circulation and in retaining the pregnancy. Zinc is also lacking in many modern diets and is necessary for a healthy pregnancy. If necessary, zinc and vitamin E supplement can be bought in health-food shops and some chemists.

3. Due to pollution and the restricted diet of many farmed animals, some authorities are recommending pregnant women to eat less meat, especially offal, but to have more white fish, free-range poultry, grains, and pulses, which are likely to be less polluted. There is also some evidence that red meat should be avoided by women suffering from high blood pressure. (Vegetable sources can provide the iron not found in white meat.)

4. Restriction of dietary salt, and iron supplementation by tablets, are controversial issues.

Additional advice to vegetarians

Anyone cutting out meat and fish from the diet can obtain adequate protein from other sources (see lists below). Be sure to eat a variety of foods at each meal in order to combine the elements that make up complete protein. If you also do not eat dairy produce, you must be particularly careful to obtain essential nutrients by eating unrefined foods, plenty of green vegetables, and dried apricots and prunes, and it is advisable to take a supplement of complete vitamin B. Addresses of vegetarian and vegan societies are given at the end of the book, should you require further information.

Coping with problems

Weight   During pregnancy the body's metabolism changes and some women put on a lot more weight than others. Whilst it is dangerous to starve yourself, there is no sense in gorging yourself. If you are worried about too great a weight gain, cut down on fats and refined carbohydrates, including sweets, and try nibbling fresh fruit and vegetables, rather than biscuits and cakes. If you like sugar in tea and coffee, limit your intake of these drinks. As an alternative, have water, or yeast or meat extract, fresh fruit juice, or herb teas, which can be made simply and cheaply by adding warm water to chopped whole fruit, or boiling water to fresh or dried herbs. If you have a good diet with adequate protein and calcium, it is unnecessary to drink extra milk.

Nausea and sickness   Many pregnant women suffer from nausea, especially in the early months. There seems to be no certain cure for it, but you may find that eating smaller meals more frequently, or having a snack before getting out of bed in the morning helps. Some people find that dry biscuits or an apple can relieve the symptoms. Avoid fat and fried foods —drinking more milk than before can also be unwise. A diet which is too high in protein and lacking carbohydrate (especially whole grains) can also cause pregnancy sickness: about one-third protein to two-thirds carbohydrate is a good balance.

Indigestion and heartburn   These can also be a nuisance in pregnancy, but don't suffer without trying to relieve them. Eat regularly, avoid large meals or going too long without food, and if certain foods cause heartburn or indigestion cut them out. Avoid sitting slouched in a chair, especially after meals. If these measures are not adequate, do not buy indigestion remedies over the counter; take only those prescribed by your doctor.

Constipation The natural slowing down of your digestive process allows more time for nourishment to be absorbed for your baby, but this should not lead to troublesome constipation if you are eating foods with a high fibre content. Eat wholemeal rather than white bread and try baking with wholemeal flour. Try breakfast cereals with a lot of whole grains and bran in them. Also make sure you have plenty of fresh fruit, prunes and figs, vegetables, and drinking-water. At least one raw meal a day is helpful.

Other advice during pregnancy

In general follow your appetite but with moderation. You may find yourself craving foods during this time of change in the body's chemistry, but try to vary your diet as much as possible anyway. If your cravings include sweet things, try eating a handful of nuts and raisins, or a piece of fresh fruit, instead of sweets or cakes.

Alcoholic drinks should be avoided as alcohol crosses the placenta and can affect the baby.

Cut out smoking or cut down to an absolute minimum. It is known to reduce the size of your baby and adversely affect his health, and therefore his chances of survival. It also destroys vitamins B and C, and zinc.

Take special care of your teeth. Pregnancy gingivitis can be avoided by gentle, regular, systematic brushing and cutting down on sugar and also on added salt (for example crisps, nuts). Tooth decay is caused by maternal neglect, not by calcium loss.

Take no medicines or drugs whatever, unless your doctor specifically tells you to.

If your cooking facilities are limited you can still eat well: muesli or other wholegrain cereals, fruit, cheese, yoghurts, wholewheat bread, and salads need no cooking. Casseroles and small pot-roasts can be cooked with vegetables in the same container—you could cook enough for two days at the same time when you feel the need of a hot meal. Good fresh food at home will help to balance the less good food which you may get if you need to eat out.

Sources of nourishment

- *Protein*   Essential for building and repairing body tissues.
    Sources: meat, poultry, fish roe;
    cheese, cottage cheese, milk, eggs, yoghurt;
    peas, beans, lentils, soya beans;
    nuts, sesame and sunflower seeds;
    flour, wheatgerm, brown rice, whole barley, wholewheat bread.
    Pulses balanced with grains make first-class protein.

- *Carbohydrates*   For energy.
    Sources: flour, bread, rice, breakfast cereals (preferably all unrefined);
    root vegetables, potatoes, peas, bananas.

- *Fats*   In moderation, for warmth and energy.
    Sources: meat, including poultry;
    herring, pilchards, sardines, sprats;
    butter, cheese, milk, eggs, margarine, lard and oils;
    nuts;
    vegetable oils, which are rich in essential fatty acids needed to limit the formation of cholesterol.

- *Minerals*
    Calcium sources: milk, dairy products including cheese, eggs, yoghurt;
    wholewheat bread, soya, oatmeal, nuts, sesame seeds, tahini, treacle, white fish;
    spinach, broccoli, cabbage, swedes, turnips, cauliflower;
    and to a lesser extent some fruit, such as oranges,

raspberries, blackberries, and dried fruit.
Also found in tap-water in hard-water areas.

Iron sources: wholewheat bread, flour, wheatgerm, wholegrain breakfast cereals, soya;
eggs, pilchards, sardines;
dried fruits, berry fruits;
haricot and butter beans, lentils, parsley, water-
cress, sprouted grains and pulses;
cocoa, chocolate, black treacle, nuts;
meat, especially red meat, liver, kidneys, heart,
sweetbreads.

There are traces of other minerals in all foods and so a
varied diet ensures adequate supplies of these. There is
some suggestion that modern diets are deficient in zinc:
this is found especially in red meat, dried peas, and beans.

- *Vitamin A*   For growth in children and for the health of moist
tissues, for example eyes and lungs.
  Sources: butter, cheese, eggs, milk, fish-liver oils, oily fish,
margarine;
carrots and all green vegetables.

- *Vitamin B*   For growth of nervous system and skin, and
prevention of some kinds of anaemia; B6 for proper utilization
of protein.
  Sources: wholewheat products, pulses;
brewer's yeast and yeast extracts;
all nuts, bananas;
fresh meat;
mushrooms.

- *Vitamin C*   For strong healthy tissues, resistance to infection, and helping the absorption of iron.
  Sources: citrus fruits, berry fruits;

green vegetables (especially raw) and salad
greens, green and red peppers, tomatoes,
potatoes, parsley;
fresh orange and lemon juice, rose-hip syrup.

- *Vitamin D*   To help the body absorb and use calcium and
phosphorus (found in dairy produce, wholewheat, and
brown rice).
   Sources: sunlight;
      fish-liver oils, oily fish, margarine, eggs, butter,
      cheese;
      liver.

- *Vitamin E*   For growth, circulation, hormone pattern, and
normal reproduction.
   Sources: wheatgerm, wholegrain cereals, green leafy
      vegetables.

- *Vitamin K*   For normal clotting of the blood.
   Sources: green leafy vegetables.

The well-nourished woman is less likely to have a premature
or low-birth-weight baby because she is less vulnerable to the
effects of infection and environmental pollution. The well-
nourished baby will withstand labour better, enter the world
stronger, and suffer less from infectious illness and allergies.

Sex in pregnancy

It is only recently that people have felt free to talk about
enjoying love-making during pregnancy; before then it was a
curiously forbidden subject. It was obvious that the prospective
parents had made love in order to conceive their baby, but after
that they were expected to develop only maternal and paternal
feelings and to sublimate any sexual passion. It was hinted that
sex could even damage the baby in some undefined way. The
fact that mothers and fathers are also lovers was glossed over.

Nowadays light is being shed on this taboo. It has its origins deep in history when, for instance, hunters, fishermen, or warriors were expected to abstain from sex before important ventures; when pregnant women were thought of as unclean and threatening, or so sacred that they were inviolable. It was also believed that pregnant women were in a state of transition between maidenhood and motherhood and were thus vulnerable. These superstitious feelings sometimes manifest themselves today in areas where good luck must be courted—many sportsmen abstain from sex before important competitions in the belief that this will somehow conserve their strength and not 'waste vital forces' in ejaculation. One could be forgiven for thinking that there is something physically or morally wrong in making love in pregnancy.

A relaxed attitude

Affectionate, tender, and spontaneous lovemaking, and the total release of orgasm, will show couples how naturally they can achieve relaxation. Many people, contemplating antenatal courses which teach relaxation exercises, feel that there is some special athleticism involved and doubt the ability of their own bodies to achieve this state: in fact, complete relaxation in a labour which is going well is, for many women, very much like relaxation after lovemaking when one feels release, calm, and emotional warmth. After the culmination of a satisfying labour and delivery women can experience an emotional 'high' akin to the deep peace which follows the most moving orgasm. The look a man sees on his partner's face after orgasm may also be there when she is enjoying her labour—her skin glows, her cheeks are flushed, her eyes shine, her hair is damp and untidy, and they both have a sense of deep satisfaction. Lovemaking and birth are both experiences which focus our attention upon the quiet centre in ourselves—and both can be upset by inhibitions or outside distractions.

Adjustments

Pregnancy can be a time of sexual discovery. Freedom from the trappings and considerations of contraception may have a liberating effect. There can be a feeling of great pride in your achievement, often mingled with ambivalence and disbelief at times, but your lovemaking has created something wonderful and each time you come together may be felt as a celebration. The powerful protective instinct often aroused in both partners can cause a change in behaviour, perhaps bringing a new gentleness to loveplay. As the baby grows and its movements are more evident, the sense of wonder increases. The gradual increase in the size of the woman's belly may have a sensual and erotic effect on the one hand and may bring a great sense of comedy and the ridiculous on the other. Devising ways of making intercourse possible in the later weeks can bring a welcome light-heartedness to your relationship, which could be a necessary preparation for the future when trying to make love with interruptions from other members of the family.

While some couples find they are more interested in sex during their pregnancy, others find the opposite is true. Sometimes the lack of interest is a mutual feeling—a quiet assent to the changes taking place in the woman's body, allowing the relationship to flourish on a more spiritual plain. Problems may arise when either partner finds that the normally pleasurable feelings aroused by sexual contact are absent, or that the contact is actually undesirable. Perhaps an orgasm is elusive, leading to feelings of frustration and hurt. It can be puzzling and confusing to be told 'I just don't fancy it', and difficult to understand why one's partner cannot even at least manage some cuddling and caressing. The growing baby may be perceived as a little invader and the enlarging abdomen viewed with dismay. Many women feel sick and lethargic in the early months and as the pregnancy progresses, the physical and emotional changes may occupy all her energies. It can be very difficult for both partners to adjust to these changes, and the isolation caused by a failure to communicate may be damaging to the relationship. A sharing of feelings and a mutual search for ways to overcome any difficulties can strengthen ties and deepen understanding.

Making love

You will find that the sheer physical changes caused by pregnancy make it necessary to adapt your technique. The 'missionary' position, with the man on top, is very uncomfortable for a pregnant woman with a bulging abdomen and sensitive, full breasts. It can be achieved with the aid of pillows under her head and shoulders, but may still induce heartburn and discomfort from deep penetration. (A few extra pillows acquired in pregnancy will also be useful for support during breastfeeding afterwards.)

Try side-to-side positions with the woman supported by pillows if her abdomen is very large. She can also kneel astride her sitting partner so that she can control the depth of penetration and he can stimulate her breasts at the same time. When the baby's head is engaged, the wife can try kneeling, crouching or lying so that her partner enters her vagina from behind. The uterus will then be virtually free from pressure since it lies almost at right angles to the vagina (see p. 6). Keeping the accent on 'making love', pregnancy is a marvellous time for discovering the joys of massage. Using an expensive massage oil, or ordinary vegetable oil, the couple can give each other great pleasure and a feeling of well-being by using simple massage techniques. Many of these will probably be a tremendous aid to pain relief during labour.

If pregnancy is advanced it may be more comfortable for the woman if her partner departs from the classic idea of ejaculation after, or during, her orgasm. There may not be enough room in the tissues of the pelvic floor for her to contain the erect penis and also do the necessary pelvic thrusts which culminate in her orgasm. Experiment with the man ejaculating first and then bringing his partner to orgasm afterwards.

The pregnant woman may find her extra-sensitive breasts an unexpected bonus, since they will be particularly responsive to her partner's touch and oral caresses. Indeed, this is a most pleasurable and effective way of preparing the nipples for breastfeeding (see p. 78).

Avoiding miscarriage

Medical opinion differs over the question of sex in relation to miscarriage. If you have already lost a baby in early pregnancy, you will probably feel very cautious anyway, and many doctors advise that intercourse should be avoided during those weeks when a period would have been due (usually only during the first three months). Massage and stimulation by touching can help to keep you physically close and satisfied during these times.

At the very end of pregnancy, if the baby is ready to be born, labour can sometimes be started by making love. This would be far pleasanter than having a drip or a cervical sweep. 'Smooching', caressing and stimulating the nipples, can certainly encourage flagging contractions during labour and is worth trying before resorting to chemical means.

Antenatal preparation for labour

We have already discussed the importance of attending an antenatal clinic to check on your own and your baby's physical states. Naturally you will also feel eager for information about pregnancy, labour, and the first weeks of life, and what you can do to help yourself through these stages. You will probably become curious about current practices in local hospitals and current ideas about what might be 'best' for the baby and for you. Hospitals do vary in their attitudes towards many aspects of the conduct of labour and postnatal care. We hope your interest will lead you to enlist in really good antenatal classes, where not only will you learn about the physiological development of your baby and what to expect during labour, but you will also have the chance to discuss and share your feelings about the whole event and share other people's feelings and ideas.

At antenatal classes you will be helped to cope with any

current problems you have and encouraged to practise further types of relaxation and breathing which can assist you during your actual labour. The easiest way to learn is from a teacher, but the following information should help those who cannot get to a class and will act as an *aide-mémoire* for those who can. Unfortunately it is not so easy to toss ideas around on paper as it is in a class discussion, and descriptions of things which are simple in demonstration can become unwieldy and pedantic in print. Please bear in mind that this chapter is intended to give you *ideas*, not a set of *rules*.

The first stage of labour

This is the time during which the uterus is pulling up and stretching the cervix over the baby's head, whilst pushing the baby lower down in the pelvis.

Early-labour breathing If you are able to have an active, ambulant labour (when you are free to walk about and to choose your own comfortable positions for each contraction), then your breathing will probably adjust itself automatically to your needs. However, if your labour is long and trying, or you need technological help (for example you have a drip, or are electronically monitored in bed), you will probably find that you need to think about the way that you are breathing and check that it is calm and rhythmical. If you have an earphone available so that no one else is disturbed, you may find listening to music helps you to relax. If the contractions become really painful and overpowering, you could try increasing the volume as a method of pain relief. However, if music, relaxation, or other aids do not help, perhaps you should discuss using analgesic drugs.

Suppose a contraction is starting. Breathe out—a long slow breath. Then gently breathe in, filling your chest as though smelling a beautiful perfume, let the air out again, and pause. Repeat this throughout the imagined contraction. As you continue to breathe regularly, check that your upper-chest and tummy muscles are relaxed; the movement of your lungs is noticeable at the lower part of your chest. Check through the rest of your body as well: feet and legs, hands and arms, shoulders and face, seat and pelvic-floor muscles—they all need to be relaxed. It can be very comforting if your partner gently massages your forehead, stroking up and out to the sides of the temple—perhaps using a cold wet cloth if you are very hot.

Practise breathing through a slightly open mouth with your lower jaw relaxed (perhaps with the beginning of a smile). This can contribute to relaxation of the vagina, which can then expand easily as the baby is pressed downwards.

Later first-stage breathing   Towards the end of the first stage you may find that lighter, slightly faster breathing is more helpful to you during contractions. You can practise this initially by balancing a small feather or a piece of tissue on the back of your hand. Lift your hand level with and near your mouth and breathe at the feather or paper, but so gently that it hardly moves on your hand. Remember to pause between breaths. Continue to start and finish each contraction with a deeper breath, and a smile. This 'resting' or finishing breath means that each contraction ends in a relaxed way.

Imagine welcoming the stronger contractions because these are the ones that will shorten your labour. These later first-stage contractions may be very difficult to cope with but remind yourself that they are the really worthwhile ones which will be dilating the cervix most effectively.

Positions in labour

In the upright position gravity helps the contractions of the uterus to press the baby's head down on the cervix, dilating it more quickly and evenly. If you lie on your back, the baby's head is not pressing down on the cervix and your labour may be slower. Lying on your back also means that the heavy uterus is pressing on the big blood vessels and slowing the circulation, which may make you feel very faint and can also lessen the baby's oxygen supply.

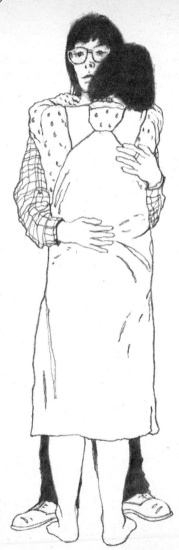

Standing

Positions you might like to consider

Standing, leaning on a window-sill or the side of the bed or trolley.

On a mattress on the floor, kneeling, resting your upper body across your companion's lap as he sits on a chair: he could massage your back in this position.

Sitting on an upright chair, leaning against its back, or leaning forward on to another surface.

Sitting astride a narrow-seated chair the wrong way round, facing its back and leaning forwards on to a pillow.

Standing with a helper, your arms round his/her neck, your head resting on his/her shoulder; your partner steadies your upper back with one hand and massages your lower back with the other.

Kneeling in bed, on all fours, or with your elbows supported on a pillow on the bed trolley, or bedhead.

Sitting upright in bed leaning forward on to the bed trolley.

Perhaps, in the event, you will feel the need to be reclining in your bed; so try lying propped up on your side (preferably your

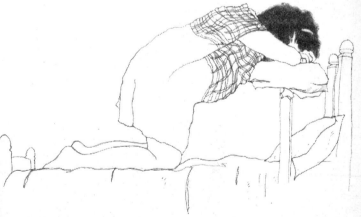

Kneeling

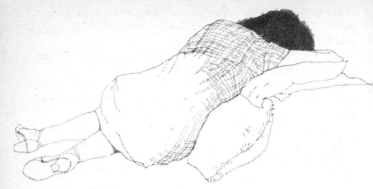

Practising side-lying

left), with your underneath arm resting up over the pillows. Experiment until you feel comfortable.

Transition phase of labour

This is the term given to the change-over from first to second stage of labour: if you have been able to maintain an upright position during the first stage, you may not be aware of an identifiable 'transition phase'. However, you may feel sick, shivery, very cross, or tearful; there may be a broken pattern of contractions which takes your breath away and makes you feel panicky. You may feel you cannot cope any more—that you want to go home and you don't want the baby anyway! The contractions may be very painful. If you feel like this you will probably be near the end of the first stage. Ask to be examined before accepting any analgesia. You may find you want to push suddenly during a contraction, but the midwife, after examining you, may tell you to wait a little longer until your cervix is fully dilated. If the cervix stretches unevenly it will leave a 'rim' or 'lip' below one part of the baby's head, although the rest of it is freed. It is like pulling a tight polo-necked sweater over your head and getting it partially stuck. The cervix will probably dilate fully if you change your position to lean towards the 'rim' of cervix that remains—your midwife can tell you which way to move. Pushing too soon against any remaining 'lip' might damage the cervix.

You may find the following suggestions helpful in controlling any feeling of panic or of wanting to push too soon.

Blow out, a short brisk breath, as if blowing a fly off the end of your nose or blowing hair out of your eyes. This releases the throat and lifts the diaphragm so that you cannot push.

Then use a repeated pattern of four light breaths: three light breaths in and out, with a light, crisp blow out on the fourth.

You may find concentrating on a phrase is helpful, for example:

Now I must blow

or

I will not push

Mouth each individual word (not the whole phrase) on a breath out. Remember to pause between breaths.

Alternatively, count on each breath out:

1 2 3 Blow

You may prefer to visualize your breaths out: bursting soap bubbles, gently, as they float past one by one. Remember the point of this is to keep your breathing calm and regular.

Or try slow, rhythmic panting as an alternative to the four-breath pattern.

You may find that it helps to make some small sound as you breathe out.

The breathing can be done into your hands cupped over your mouth and nose. This makes a noise for you to listen to and also helps to prevent overbreathing (hyperventilation), which can make you feel dizzy or give you cramp, and is not good for your baby.

Other aids during transition

You may find that calm breathing combined with controlled activity helps you to cope with this phase. The activities could be any of the following, so bear them all in mind when you are 'rehearsing' antenatally:

- Massaging your lower back, or massaging your thighs, or massaging round or under the 'bump' (your partner could do any of these for you).
- Gently bulging your tummy muscles forward by pressure from your hands placed on either side of the bump.
- Tapping your fingers in a rhythm (your arm should be supported so that only your fingers and hand move), mouthing the words of a song you have chosen, or counting backwards. Concentrating on this mouthing may help to distract you from the strength of the contraction and your breathing will be automatically corrected.
- Using gas and oxygen (Entonox) will help to counteract the urge to push, but note that there is a delay between inhaling Entonox and its having an effect, and similarly its effect lasts after your last breath of it. It also becomes more effective once there is a little in the bloodstream, so that even if your first attempt to use it seems ineffectual, it is worth persevering for a few contractions. The art is to inhale just in advance of the start of the contraction and then leave the mask off whilst you are coping with the contraction, after which you will have time to return to a sufficiently alert state to start using the mask effectively before the next contraction becomes established. You need to put your hand on your bump (or ask your partner to do this for you) to feel the very first signs of the uterus starting to tighten; at that point take, say, four deep but not too leisurely breaths of Entonox, which will take you over the peak of the contraction. If your labour is being electronically monitored you will be able to see from the readings on the screen the early indications of a coming contraction; or simply timing the intervals between contractions may help.
- Should you need it, Entonox can be used throughout labour.
- Sucking a mouthful of crushed ice, sucking on a small natural sponge, or spraying your face with 'fizzy' water (soda or mineral) from a small plastic bottle can be very refreshing. A

frozen picnic-pack, or ice-pack, put on your back can relieve aching.

- Maintaining eye contact with your partner.
- Reminding yourself that you are very nearly ready to push.
- At this stage you may have only half a minute's rest between contractions, which may last perhaps a minute and a half. In between contractions try to relax completely and catnap. If you have to be moved to a different room at this time you may find that the move interferes with your contractions and they may stop completely for a short while. Enjoy the rest, knowing that the contractions will start again before too long.

Examination during transition

If, at the time, you are sitting or on your side: rock yourself back so that the lower part of your back is against the bed, but your head and shoulders are well propped up against the pillows. If

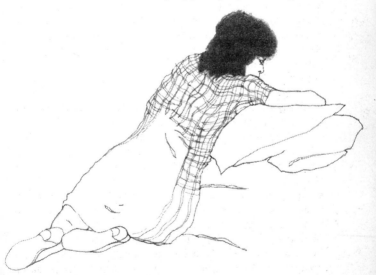

Practising sitting on one side

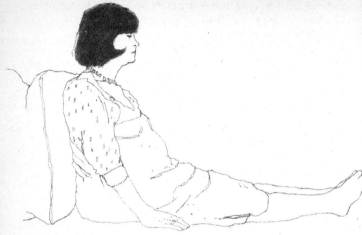

Sitting upright

you are in a kneeling position, the midwife may be able to examine you if you stay there. Whatever your position, let your pelvic floor relax as her fingers feel the baby's head. If she says that the baby is not completely through the cervix you may find that a position (illustrated below) on your knees and elbows for

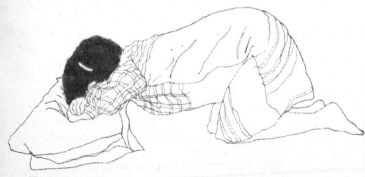

On knees and elbows

a few contractions helps the baby to rotate into a better position. You should get help to change your position.

The second stage of labour

The second stage is the time after the cervix is fully dilated until the birth of the baby. Sometimes there is a quiet period before the pushing urge begins. Take advantage of the opportunity to rest, as mentioned above. The uterus will do the greater part of the pushing, to get the baby through the birth canal, but you can work with it in a positive way. Most women find this part really satisfying.

Positions for the second stage

If this is your first baby, it isn't easy to imagine how you will feel at the time. Try out the following ideas when you are practising antenatally: some positions may already seem more likely to you than others, but of course when you are in labour your baby will be in a different position from the one it is in now. The important thing is to realize that you have the freedom to choose positions and to change positions.

Some women prefer to stand—well supported—to push. If you choose this position let your weight be taken completely by your helper: his/her arms under your arms and his/her fingers linked tightly across your upper chest, your body supported against their body. As you bear down, your knees will bend a little so that you are in a semi-squatting position. It is unnecessary to squat right down on your heels and it may make the birth more difficult if you do.

Some hospitals are now providing birth chairs to support you in a more upright sitting position during your labour and delivery. If your hospital has a large or a small chair do ask to try it, preferably early in your labour so that you have time to make yourself comfortable. If, however, it does not seem to help you, ask to change position—either move on to a bed or perhaps stand on a mattress on the floor.

One of the small plastic boxes sold for children to stand on at the wash-basin may be found helpful as a birth stool. They are

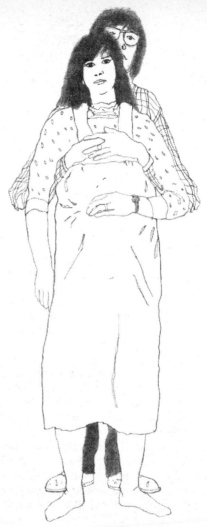

Standing, well supported

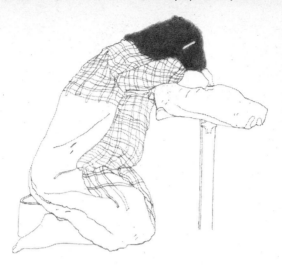

Using a birth stool

kidney shaped with a continuous base, and being only about 6 inches high can be used on a bed, or on a mattress, or clean sheet, on the floor. Your partner could support you from behind.

If you think you might prefer to sit on a bed, or mattress, practise sitting not on your bottom but rocked back on the base of your spine with your back and shoulders well supported (as illustrated). You should have your knees bent and feet well apart. Let your legs flop apart so that the outer edges of your feet rest on the bed. Putting your hands round your legs in front of your knees helps you to feel stable on the bed. It may be better if you sit slightly sideways (on one buttock) with one knee bent up and the other leg relaxed on the bed (see illustration); or you may like to start pushing in a kneeling position or on all fours and perhaps turn and sit for the actual birth.

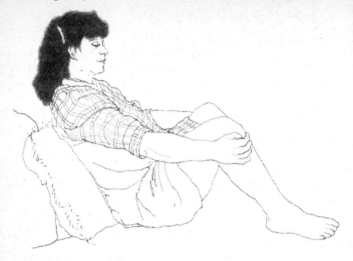

Sitting, rocked back on base of spine

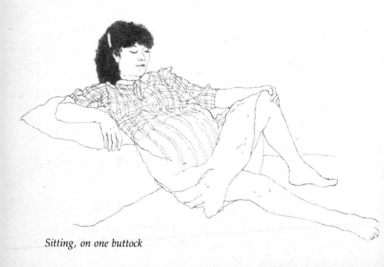

Sitting, on one buttock

Breathing for the second stage

Many women find that their breathing adapts itself automatically and that they are breathing and pushing quite spontaneously. There is no advantage to be gained from prolonged pushing and breath-holding. Hold your breath for short periods, and push your diaphragm down (as though you were doing a silent cough) to help you guide your baby down and forward out of the birth canal. Follow the pattern set by your body. Remember the importance of being comfortably upright so that gravity helps the baby out. The following suggestions may help you to work with your body.

As you imagine the contraction starting, breathe out, breathe in, out, and pause.

Breathe in and tilt your head forward so that you lean down on the baby (feel that the weight of your head, arms, and chest is bearing down through your body).

Continue to breathe as you need. You may need to hold your breath during each wave of pushing which occurs during each contraction. Alternatively you may like to try blowing out slowly and firmly with each pushing urge. As you blow out you will feel the muscles round your waist tightening: this helps to move your baby down. Remember to pause between breaths.

Let your pelvic floor relax as the baby bulges it outwards and you give birth.

Remember to have your mouth slightly open so that it is relaxed, which in turn should help your vagina to relax also.

You may find yourself making a noise as you push.

Between contractions relax and breathe normally.

If you do not develop the urge to push, try kneeling or a supported squat during contractions.

If you remain unaware of an urge to push, ask the midwife to guide you.

The delivery of your baby

As your baby is being born, the midwife may tell you to stop pushing: blow out, relax your pelvic floor, and then breathe lightly with your mouth slightly open. Remember to pause between breaths. This requires very gentle panting breathing, which you will continue to do until the midwife tells you to push again. You may be aware of a fleeting burning sensation before your baby's head 'crowns'.

As the baby slides out you may feel the ridges of eyebrows, nose, cheek-bones, and chin as they slide over the back of your birth canal. Usually the uterus rests before it contracts again to deliver the shoulders and the rest of the baby's body. You may like to touch your baby's head during this time, in welcome. This skin contact between the two of you can speed up the next contraction, which will free the baby from the pressure of the birth canal and help him/her to breathe. Remember to relax your mouth as the shoulders are born—you will probably be smiling at your baby anyway.

Variations in the second stage

If you need assistance for the baby's birth your legs will probably be supported in stirrups and you will be asked not to push until the doctor has applied his fingers, or the forceps, or the vacuum cap (for a Ventouse delivery) on to the baby's head. You will still need your head and shoulders well propped up and you can ask the doctor to tell you when you can start to push again, in the manner already described, so that you can help to deliver your baby.

If the baby is in the breech position (bottom first instead of head first) the same applies, although you will probably be able to push your baby's legs and body out before you have assistance to deliver his/her head.

If there are not enough pillows on the bed and there is no one who can support you (your partner could sit on the bed behind you so that you can lean against him), prop yourself well up on your elbows. This will round your shoulders and tilt your head towards your chest.

Third stage of labour

This is the delivery of the placenta (afterbirth) and it usually happens quite soon after the baby is born. You may be asked to push or cough to help the placenta to slide out of the birth canal.

Points to remember

There is no special depth at which you should be breathing. This will vary according to your position and that of your baby, how relaxed you are and how strong the contraction is at the time.

Your breathing rate should be one which is comfortable for you—neither too slow nor too fast. You should feel that you could continue to breathe in that particular way for as long as necessary. Use deeper or lighter breathing to help you find your own way of coping with each different stage of labour.

If you feel giddy or light-headed, with numbness or tingling around your mouth or in your fingers, it means that you are over-breathing. Should this happen, breathe into your cupped hands, check that your breathing is not too vigorous, and remember to pause between breaths. Then sit yourself up more, keeping your back straight, or stand up and lean forward on to something. This will help to regularize and calm your breathing, and relieve the pressure on your diaphragm.

In the second stage there should be effort but no undue strain—usually there is no hurry or urgency. Follow the pattern set by your body; remember the importance of being comfortably upright so that gravity helps the baby out.

If you are anxious about how you will cope with pain in labour, two realistic thoughts may help you.

You could remind yourself that your tissues are designed to be tight enough to support the weight of the growing baby, the placenta, and the liquor. Obviously this means that stretching and therefore some pain will be inevitable as the birth canal opens up to let the baby be born.

You may find it helpful to recall that pain is often associated with extra effort which people demand from themselves: the even further stretch made by the ballet dancer; the even greater pace achieved by the sprinter in order to beat his own record; the extra effort we've all put in at some time, when our muscles were telling us to stop digging/polishing/decorating but we pushed ourselves to complete the task to our satisfaction.

Emotional preparation for parenthood

Pregnancy is a perfectly normal state for a woman to be in, but it is also a time of mental and physical adjustment, just like any other major change in your life. Your emotional responses to the pregnancy are just as important as the physical changes you are experiencing: you may, for instance, become suddenly aware of all the responsibility you have taken on, not only for the development of your baby before it is born, but also for the care and raising of a child which will be dependent on you for many years to come. Or you may find yourself swamped by such variety of advice and such a mass of choices that you do not know where to turn, because what seemed so simple— to have a baby—now involves all kinds of uncertainties you had not anticipated. Fortunately the nine months of gestation give you plenty of time in which to prepare to be a parent— it doesn't happen overnight. And it may be comforting to remind yourself that the baby will also be a first-timer and will not be comparing your efforts at parenting with anyone else's!

Pregnancies are very different experiences for different people. Some people are delighted to be pregnant, others are not pleased at all, still others accept the situation without great emotion either way. Some women find that pregnancy makes them feel unwell or ungainly, other women feel that they have never been healthier, and yet others cope with some discomforts and inconveniences but enjoy some benefits as well. Some couples find that pregnancy is a welcome and positive extension of their marriage; others find it a strain on their relationship, whether or not the baby was planned. Your pregnancy will be unlike anyone else's and will depend more on your personality than on anyone else's experience. It is best to take your pregnancy as it comes, neither counting on storybook bliss nor expecting the worst to happen.

When you do have bad days—and they come to virtually everyone at some point—try to find something really enjoyable to do as compensation and don't let yourself be led into thinking that the discouragement or discomfort will necessarily continue or that there is no solution. Treating yourself to whatever seems a self-indulgent pleasure in the circumstances will often have a restorative effect: if you are at home, put the chores aside and curl up in an armchair to read, do some fancy cooking, go for a walk, or invite a neighbour in for a cup of coffee; if you are at work, look forward to a long lazy bath when you reach home, have something special for lunch, get some fresh air during a break, or have a cup of tea (special flavoured teas and herbal teas may be particularly refreshing). If you feel like it, decide on the spur of the moment to do something special with your husband—maybe there is a film you have been wanting to see—or, on the other hand, allow yourself to decline invitations if you feel too tired to socialize.

When a pregnancy is confirmed, a woman's body suddenly becomes the subject of unblushing attention, with everyone —doctor and midwife, colleagues, family, and neighbours— talking freely about how well or tired she is looking, what and how much she should or should not eat, how big or how small her abdomen is, what exercise she should or should not take, and so forth. The feeling that the pregnancy which you thought was a private and loving affair between you and your partner is now a matter for public discussion can be very upsetting, and it is easy to resent the feeling that people seem to treat you as if you no longer had any interests other than the baby and indeed were important only because of the baby. Even if you faithfully attend your regular antenatal checks, and recognize their importance in ensuring your health and the baby's, you may feel that all this attention invades your privacy, questions your ability to take care of yourself, and implies that your body is no longer your own but belongs to the clinic, or the doctor, or the baby, more than to yourself.

Pregnancy involves so many changes that it is not surprising that it takes some time to adjust to the idea. Just as starting a new job often raises doubts about whether you have made the right choice until you have settled in, so starting a family may give you some second thoughts. This is perfectly natural. At some point in pregnancy practically every woman wishes she had never embarked on the adventure. For most, this is only a temporary feeling, but for some it lasts throughout the pregnancy and colours the entire experience.

The woman who resents pregnancy

Some women simply do not like being pregnant. It may be that pregnancy makes the woman feel physically unwell, although she wants the baby, or it may be that she really does not want to have a baby at all, for whatever reason: perhaps she had planned a career which just does not fit in with being a mother; perhaps her personal circumstances have changed so that she wishes she had never become pregnant; perhaps the pregnancy was unplanned and came as an unwanted upset to the couple's expectations. If she has always been super-efficient she may hate the forgetfulness that so often comes with pregnancy; if she is accustomed to subduing her body to her intellectual needs or to pressures of work she may resent the tiredness and digestive demands of pregnancy; if she has led an active social life she may dread that pregnancy will make her feel or be unattractive and that having a baby will put an end to her freedom.

When a woman like this first realizes that she is pregnant, she may become extremely depressed and consider abortion, or she may refuse to accept that she is pregnant, but as time passes and her labour seems far ahead she may get used to the idea. When her 'bump' starts to show she may go through another bad patch—perhaps wearing a tight girdle to flatten her abdomen or starving herself in the hope that if she becomes thin she will not look pregnant. Perhaps the worst time is when she finally gives up work and begins to feel trapped at home. Her antenatal appointments become more frequent, she is offered antenatal classes, and everyone around her not only seems to be conspiring to remind her that soon she will be a mother, but also assumes that she is delighted at the prospect. She may easily decide to opt out of experiencing her labour by requesting an induction-and-epidural package, letting the machines and the doctor do everything so that she is minimally involved. (Of course, not every woman who seeks the help of medical technology during childbirth is 'opting out'—sometimes a woman will need an epidural to make her birth safer.)

This is painting the blackest picture and no one person is likely to go through all these negative stages; but it would be unrealistic and unwise to pretend that pregnancy automatically brings bliss, or that motherhood automatically means joy. Dreamy fantasies portrayed in advertisements bear little relation to the way most people feel and live.

To counteract these gloomy possibilities the frustrated career woman needs to use her intellect to make a career out of her pregnancy and motherhood. You may find comfort during your pregnancy by enquiring into the chances of either taking the baby to work with you or finding a registered baby-minder. The same applies of course to the woman who needs to work for financial reasons. If your job is not physically demanding, you may be able to continue with your work throughout your pregnancy. If you feel forced by the pressures of your family or neighbours to stay at home with your baby, this could have an adverse effect on your feelings towards the child; it is far better to find some way of returning to a job if that is what *you* need to do and then you may be able to be your own kind of 'good mother' and enjoy your child during the times between work. However, it is important that the baby has a constant caretaker and is not passed around to just any willing person.

The local county social services department is a good source of information about registered child-minders. For information about financial allowances you should consult the Department of Health and Social Security.

The changing hormone pattern during pregnancy can be a cause of mood swings, but they are not an excuse for constant bad temper and general dissatisfaction. Set about coping with pregnancy in a sensible manner: inform yourself about aspects of pregnancy, labour, and motherhood—and in particular take care of your diet. If you eat correctly you should feel and look well, the minor ills of pregnancy will be minimized, and the baby's growth and development will be helped.

Further observations

So far we have considered the difficulties of the woman who wishes she were not pregnant, but even the woman who is overjoyed to find herself pregnant may have problems. You may have periods of excessive tiredness, of feeling sick, or apparently unaccountable depression or anxiety. If you are eating correctly and getting an adequate amount of rest and exercise but still feeling low, you may like to add a vitamin E supplement to your diet. This will help the hormone balance and improve the condition of the placenta. The woman who becomes severely depressed or who habitually miscarries about the third to fourth month of pregnancy may be helped by progesterone therapy prescribed by her doctor. This usually involves a course of injections. Some women feel well if they take extra iron and vitamin B. In all of these cases, however, consult your doctor.

The woman who is fit and happy during her pregnancy is likely to transmit her confidence and well being to her partner so that he may share with her the joyful reality of pregnancy and anticipation of parenthood. She is likely to glow with health, to be keen to work with her body in adapting to pregnancy and coping with labour, and to be excited at the prospect of seeing her own baby.

Pregnancy can be a trying time for an expectant father, who may have just as many anxieties as his wife. Will the baby be normal? Might I lose my job and not be able to support my wife and child financially? If my wife becomes depressed during pregnancy will she ever return to normal? And so on. The man and woman may need to reassure and support each other. It is a good idea for *both* parents to inform themselves about the baby's growth and development and what happens to the mother during pregnancy, and the same applies to labour and parenthood. If you have anxieties which cannot be cleared up in antenatal classes or by reading, you could go together to the antenatal clinic so that there are two of you to ask the questions, and to make sure that you see a sufficiently senior member of the staff until you have answers which satisfy and reassure you. Discuss beforehand the gist of what you want to say and what you want to find out, and remember that should a choice be necessary, you can go away to discuss the matter by yourselves and return later to the doctor to let him know your decision. It is likely to be difficult to talk with the doctor if you are lying undressed on the examination couch, so ask the doctor if you can see him again when you are dressed to discuss his recommendations.

Nowadays men and women are able to choose when and if they will have children, and this makes it a natural step for them to want to take responsibility for the health of the mother and the baby during pregnancy and to give the baby as well prepared and gentle a birth as possible. Some couples have found it helpful to write a 'Birth Plan': a list of things they would especially like to happen during labour and the subsequent hospital stay. This can be discussed with the doctor and mid-wife at the antenatal clinic and a copy put in your notes. It is not a good idea to hand it over during labour. Keep a copy to take into hospital with you to jog your own memory. It could cover such points as the use of technology in labour, your views on drugs (including Syntometrine), birth positions, and care of the baby, and also making the point that you realize that modifica-tion may be necessary if the labour is not straightforward. With this in mind we suggest you read the section beginning on p. 99 so that you can think ahead on these issues and you should also note our further reading list (p. 289).

The advantages of breastfeeding

One of the things you and your husband should think about before your baby is born is whether you want to breastfeed. Breastfeeding is so good for the baby that you should consider giving it a try—at the very least while you are in hospital, for it will give the baby protection from the germs he will meet there. If you continue for four to six months your baby will have had the best possible start. Some mothers and babies are happy to continue for much longer.

Most breastfeeding failures arise from lack of information. There are many myths about breastfeeding, and there are also many facts which you can learn beforehand about the advantages of natural feeding and about how your breasts function. In this way you will understand what is happening and will be able to differentiate between good and bad advice. It will also give you calmness and self-confidence, which are very important.

Breastfeeding is fashionable again after a time when bottle-feeding was the norm. Some nurses and midwives who trained during the time when artificial feeding predominated may not be used to giving breastfeeding help and may pay lip service to it while unintentionally giving inaccurate advice. So learn enough during pregnancy to be your own counsel when the baby arrives. Of course, if problems occur that you cannot cope with, you can always get in touch with your doctor, your health visitor, or your local NCT breastfeeding counsellor, who has been trained by the Breastfeeding Promotion Group of the NCT to give advice on practical, non-medical, breastfeeding problems.

Some good reasons for breastfeeding

Midwives and doctors agree that breast milk is the perfect first food for babies. Its constituents are quite different in their proportions from cows' milk, which has to be extensively modified in order to make it suitable for human babies. It is more difficult for the kidneys of young babies to excrete the extra mineral salts found in artificial milks.

Colostrum, the high-protein fluid which precedes breast milk proper, is particularly valuable. It contains antibodies to many of the diseases you have had or have been immunized against and helps protect against the bacteria which cause gastro-enteritis. The risk of gastro-enteritis is much greater in bottle-fed babies, especially where bottle sterilization is inefficient.

There is a certain amount of evidence that breastfed babies seem less likely to develop allergies such as eczema and asthma.

Breastfed babies are less likely to get fat than bottle-fed babies. Fat babies often become fat adults, and fat adults are more prone to heart disease, arterial disease, and diabetes. Fat babies are also more prone to colds and chest infections.

Breastfed babies are never constipated. Although they sometimes go for several days without a bowel motion, because breast milk is so perfectly absorbed, the stool—when it comes—is always soft. Breastfed babies' motions have a less strong smell than those produced by bottle-fed babies, because there are different fats in breast milk.

Breastfeeding helps you to get your figure back to normal more quickly. Soon after birth the hormones involved in breast-feeding cause 'afterpains' which help the uterus to contract back to its pre-pregnancy size and position. A longer period of breastfeeding uses up any extra fat which has been put on in pregnancy (for just this purpose).

Breastfeeding saves time—a valuable commodity to the new mother. Breast milk is always available, at the right temperature, when your baby is hungry. He never has to be kept waiting while you sterilize bottles or warm up feeds.

Breastfeeding is cheaper than bottle-feeding: bottles, teats, sterilizing equipment, and artificial milk all cost money. However, a breastfeeding mother needs more food for herself than a woman who is feeding her baby artificially. You may want to have a bottle and sterilizing solution available for emergencies.

Breastfeeding gives you automatic closeness to your baby. For the child, it is warmth, comfort, and food all rolled into one. For you, the mother, it is usually a very enjoyable experience.

Breast milk is a complete food for your baby for the first four to six months of life. Since the risks of ill-health are greater when the baby is very young, breastfeeding for even as little as two weeks is an advantage.

Antenatal advice about breastfeeding

Whether or not you plan to breastfeed your baby, your breasts will start preparing themselves during pregnancy. You will notice an increase in size during the first three months and will probably need a larger bra. Heavy unsupported breasts may develop stretch marks. Broad non-stretch straps will probably be most comfortable now and you should avoid underwires as they could damage the developing tissue. If your breasts are very heavy, a sleep bra or a nightie that supports the breasts could be worn at night for comfort. From the seventh month, the Mava maternity and nursing bra is very comfortable, being designed to allow for your expanding rib-cage. It is a front-opening bra: trapdoor-type nursing bras (drop-down flap) may damage the milk-producing glands (the pressure can restrict the milk flow and cause blocked ducts). The Mava bra, which comes in an exceptionally wide range of sizes, is exclusive to the NCT, being available by mail order or from agents attached to NCT branches.

Another change you will notice during pregnancy is that the little bumps on the areola (the darker skin around the nipple) become more prominent. These are glands which secrete an oily cream to keep the skin supple and elastic. It is a pity to waste this natural lubrication by vigorous washing using a lot of soap. Gentle washing and patting dry is all that is required.

Nipples are often very tender during pregnancy and rough handling will be uncomfortable. Some mothers-to-be like to apply extra oil to their breasts, especially if they have dry skin. There are special breast creams on the market, all of which are suitable, but any cream or oil which suits your skin type will do equally well. Smooth it gently into the areola and nipple once a day. Using too much is messy, wasteful, and makes the skin soggy, predisposing to soreness later on.

Your doctor or midwife should examine your breasts when feeding is discussed with you early in pregnancy. The shape and size of nipples vary and you may be wondering if yours are all right. Towards the end of pregnancy all nipples improve in the amount they stand out. A quick 'do-it-yourself' test is to press behind the areola with your finger and thumb. If the nipple stands out it will be OK for the baby. If the nipple goes inwards, it is inverted and you may like to wear breast shells to help it to come out. These can be prescribed by your doctor or midwife. Do follow carefully the instructions provided with the shells and stop using them if your nipples get sore.

After the baby is born, using a hand or electric pump before feeding may help to draw out flat nipples sufficiently for the baby to latch on. Making the nipple cold by applying ice also makes it stand out, but may be too painful to do.

Colostrum

Colostrum is a protein-enriched food which is made in the breast from the fourth month of pregnancy. Sometimes some oozes out and dries on the nipple, where you will see it as yellow crumbs. These will be washed away when you have your bath. Some breasts leak colostrum, probably because the small muscle behind the nipple is lax. This could be improved by splashing the nipples with cold water or running an ice cube around the areola. If your nipples are very tender, you will not welcome this suggestion!

Leaking colostrum can be messy and distressing. Do not worry that there will be none left for the baby. Colostrum will continue to be made while you are pregnant. Cope with the dampness by putting breast pads or folded clean hankies inside your bra. Try to avoid using plastic-backed pads as they keep the skin hot and moist and lead to soggy skin and soreness. Try to expose your breasts to the air for some time each day to help dry the skin. Minimize washing of bedclothes by putting a piece of plastic under the sheet, or lie on a towel.

If you don't see any signs of colostrum, don't worry. It is there and will be ready for your baby when he arrives. It is not necessary to express (squeeze out) colostrum during pregnancy.

For expectant fathers

Pregnancy is a time when there are significant developments which can put stress on even the happiest relationships. It is as though the invisible bonds which join a loving couple must be untied and reassembled to make that couple into a family. During pregnancy, the expectant mother usually gets a lot of support from her family and friends, from her doctor, the hospital, and her antenatal class, but the father's need for support during this maturing process is not usually recognized.

This book, and this chapter, are written to help you understand your feelings, and your partner's during her pregnancy.

Pregnancy

Many couples are torn between wanting to start a family and facing a change in their lifestyle: your partner may have to give up her job and you will have to face much greater financial responsibility. She may also miss her working friends and, while waiting for the baby to be born, find cleaning and cooking a poor substitute for the stimulus of a job outside the home.

A first pregnancy is a challenge to the couple's ability, not only to make adjustments to their way of life, but also to cope with major changes in the mother's body. During the first three months she will not look pregnant but will be acutely aware of her pregnancy from the moment it has been diagnosed. She may be sick or sleepy—or on the other hand, she may hardly have any physical symptoms. In this case she will resent being mollycoddled but should still be encouraged to rest more than usual. As the baby grows and develops, chemical changes take place stimulated by the glands which also play a part in controlling the emotions. During pregnancy most women are, therefore, much more emotionally on edge than usual. You will probably find the middle three months are a more stable period.

Try to keep up her morale during the last few weeks by finding interesting things to do together—especially if she passes her estimated date of delivery. To her, each 'extra' day will seem like an age, so be patient and understanding if she is grumpy and frustrated. She may need reassurance that you still find her attractive in spite of the bulk of her body.

Before she goes for her regular antenatal visits, talk things over so that if either of you has any queries she can make a note and ask them during her examination. You may like to accompany her and share this responsibility with her—antenatal clinics increasingly welcome the father's interest. You can help to remember the questions you both wanted to ask, help to persist in getting answers, and help to remember the information you are given. Afterwards you can remind her to carry out any particular advice she has been given and encourage her to keep to a healthy diet (see p. 42).

She will probably be invited to go to preparation classes at her hospital or local clinic, and may also wish to attend NCT classes. Encourage her to go and then to tell you the things she has learned. A woman can give birth without knowing anything about the process, but it can be very frightening and unpleasant. A good course of antenatal preparation will help her to train her mind and her body to cope with the experiences of pregnancy and labour. Attend classes with her if you can: some antenatal teachers teach couples, while others include a father's evening in the course. You will learn many interesting facts to refute the horror stories with which expectant parents are bombarded, plus hints on recognizing the onset of labour and lots of suggestions for making things easier for both of you.

Discuss beforehand whether you wish to be together during labour, and find out what steps you should take to make this possible. Slides or a film of a birth may clarify your ideas, but not everyone wants to see someone else's baby delivered before they see their own—the emotional commitment is just not comparable. Many men have a distorted idea of the amount of blood and suffering in labour and feel they would hate to witness it. They do not realize how involved they will feel inside the room, doing something helpful, rather than pacing the corridor outside. Many couples feel that sharing this experience of birth has given a deeper meaning to their relationship and to their feelings for the child. The vast majority of fathers rate it one of the most important experiences of their lives. A well-prepared father can be of assistance to the midwifery staff as well as to the mother, but you should be clear in your mind that your role will be to comfort and support your partner and help her cope with the hospital setting. Your familiar presence should act as an aid to relaxation and can help to counteract possible feelings of inhibition in the presence of hospital staff, some of whom may be complete strangers.

Long before the expected date of delivery discuss how your child will be fed. More and more women are wishing to feed their babies naturally, and reading informed facts about breast-feeding (p. 169) will help give you both confidence. A woman who cannot breastfeed her baby, for physical or emotional reasons, needs your support too. If your partner is not sure how to feed the baby, encourage her to breastfeed, at least for the first few days, when the fluid in her breasts (colostrum) is especially valuable for your baby's health and digestion.

Prelude to labour

It is wise to have everything ready for the baby three weeks before the due date. Your partner will feel happier if she has a telephone number where she can reach you during the day or, if this is not possible, the number of a friend who is willing to sit with her during early labour. Pin a list of the telephone numbers of midwives, doctors, hospital, and ambulance by your telephone. If you have no telephone, keep some coins of the right size for your local call-box in a convenient place. If you plan to drive to the hospital, check petrol and tyres regularly. Keep a couple of cushions and a rug in the car and make sure you are familiar with the best routes to the admission block, both by night and during rush hours.

If the baby is to be born at home, check your fuel supply and make sure that you have fuse-wire and an alternative source of heat for the bedroom available in winter. Some extra pillows may be required and the midwife might find a bedside lamp or powerful torch useful.

The onset of labour

You will have read about the three common signs that labour is beginning: regular contractions felt as menstrual cramp, back-ache, or wind; the 'show' or blood-streaked plug of jelly from the cervix (which may appear some days before labour is established), and the gushing or breaking of the waters. Many women, however, do not have these definite signs and it is difficult to decide when the vague intermittent sensations, which the early contractions of the uterus give rise to, are the 'real thing'. Wait until the contractions become longer, stronger, and at shorter intervals, before notifying the hospital or sending for the midwife. If the confinement is to be at home, make sure that your house is warm and well lit and that light refreshments are available. If you are going into hospital to stay with your partner, you may need warm clothing for a chilly night vigil but later be glad to strip down to a cotton shirt if you are going into the delivery room. You may like to prepare and take with you a bag containing:

- *Frozen picnic freezing bag* to put against your partner's back if she has backache.

- *Small natural sponge* to moisten her mouth and spray bottle of 'fizzy' water to cool her face.

- *Lipsalve or vaseline* to prevent her lips becoming chapped.

- *Jigsaws, books, playing cards, etc.*, in case it is a long-drawn-out labour with long gaps between contractions.
- *Vacuum flask of cracked ice* for her to suck during labour (to make it more refreshing, the ice could be made from water containing some fresh fruit juice).
- *Refreshments*—drinks, sandwiches, etc. for you, with enough left for her to have after the birth if she has just missed a hospital mealtime.
- *Change* for the hospital telephone box.
- *Small plastic box* for her to sit on.

(You should keep the bag containing these things, since your partner's belongings may be removed for safekeeping.)

Labour

You will find a clear description of the course of labour on pp. 105–12, with suggestions about how both parents can cope with the sequence of events.

As labour advances, a woman's thoughts are focused on what is happening to her body, and she has no time for the niceties of behaviour. Her emotions are near the surface and may easily spill over into laughter or tears, particularly at the moment of birth. She may swear or snap at you during the transition phase. Take it all in good part and adapt to meet her needs; you are in a better position than anyone else to do this. In a hospital, nurses have other patients and other duties to attend to, you have only your partner. If you are quiet and obviously competent, they will welcome your presence. Stand up for your partner's wishes, but do not be aggressive: this will only antagonize the staff. If you want something, be polite, but firm and confident in your requests.

When you are present at the delivery, don't be surprised if you, too, don't know whether to laugh or to cry. It is an unforgettable experience to see your newborn child come into the world. New babies may be deep pink or even purple, be wrinkled like old men, show traces of blood or the white cream which covered them while they were in the uterus, and their heads can be a peculiar shape with a bump at the back. The genitals of a newborn baby often seem unexpectedly large. If you have never seen a very young child, make a point of looking at some colour photographs of new babies. They do not look at all like the chubby, smiling cherubs in glossy advertisements.

Personal experience

A father wrote this shortly after the birth of his child:

'A postscript for future fathers

Regardless of where the baby is being born, at home or hospital, be prepared to leave your sense of embarrassment somewhere else—you will soon realize that what is happening to your wife is the most real thing she has ever experienced. She will do things which, under normal circumstances would be ludicrous, she will groan and moan softly or loudly, she may become totally uninterested in you, she will ask you questions you have no answers for ('How much longer?') . . . so, since she is putting her whole self into her labour it will help her and you if you become as totally involved as possible. You can help her greatly by answering questions the nurses ask and by making the decisions—she is in no state to think about anything but what is happening to her body. And above all, be positive. Never cast even the shadow of a doubt into her mind. Always tell her that she is doing well, because no matter what she is doing she is doing the best she can. Do not judge her—help her, give her some of your energy.

The amount of togetherness you discover during the birth of your child will remain with you and grow for the rest of your lives.'

LABOUR &
BIRTH

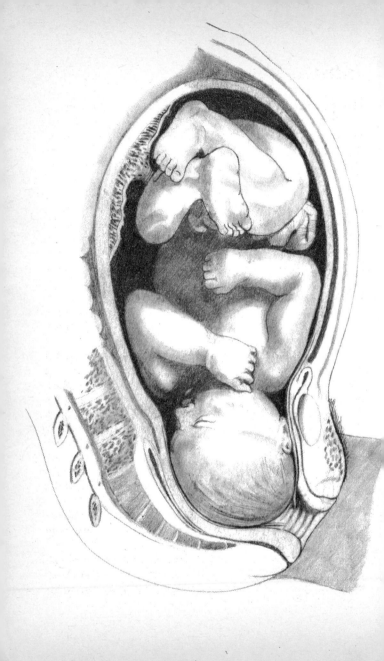

Introduction

Having a baby is hard physical work and emotionally demanding. It is possible to do it without any knowledge or training but, unless you are very lucky, the experience may be traumatic if you undergo it with no idea how to help yourself. A non-swimmer thrown into the deep end of a pool is unlikely to enjoy the experience or look back on it with much satisfaction. She will be relieved to find that she has survived and will want to forget the experience. She may be left with a fear of water, or may determine to learn to swim so that she can't be put at such a disadvantage again. A practised swimmer can have a great deal of pleasure from the challenges offered by the water and set by herself—from the physical sensations of swimming and diving. There are lots of mothers who only want to put their labours behind them and thank goodness that the baby is fine and so are they themselves. There are also lots who are pleased to recall the experience: tumultuous and challenging with amazing physical sensations.

National Childbirth Trust antenatal preparation can never guarantee you an easy birth, but it does offer confidence-giving knowledge, practical information, and a range of useful suggestions for coping with the many variations there are on the theme of giving birth. You can expect to learn in which circumstances analgesic drugs may be helpful and when they may be being offered without discrimination: timing can be all important. You will also learn which medical practices are commonly used routinely and sometimes unnecessarily, as well as learning how to co-operate with life-saving procedures should the need arise.

Your partner can learn how to be an active and useful helper during your labour, so that you may feel that you have truly shared the experience.

Though many women prefer to have their babies in hospital, you may wish to have your baby at home. For low-risk cases, this is an option to consider, provided your home conditions are suitable and there is a maternity hospital within easy reach.

Sometimes, of course, complications arise in giving birth. Some babies have to be born by Caesarean section and, if this happens, you will have to cope with post-operative pain and other discomforts as well as the usual joys and stresses of early motherhood. Many women nowadays have to cope with the pain caused by stitches in the perineum after the birth outlet has been enlarged by an incision during delivery: this is especially true for a woman having her first baby or a forceps delivery.

Medical research is now showing what ordinary mothers could have testified for generations: that uninterrupted early contact between you and your newborn baby is important for you both, and so your baby should not be separated from you at all. If either of you is ill you can make arrangements with the paediatrician so that you can still be together as much as possible.

The anatomy and physiology of labour

Labour is the process of childbirth which occurs at the end of pregnancy, usually about 40 weeks from the date of your last period. Three stages of labour can be identified, each of which has a specific function. The first stage pulls up and opens the neck of the uterus, called the cervix. The second stage is the journey of your baby along the birth canal, from the uterus to the outside world. The third stage involves the delivery of the afterbirth, or placenta, which completes the process.

The first stage

This is usually the longest part of labour, and with a first baby used to average about ten hours, but this seems to be reducing now women are being encouraged to be active and not lie in bed, and we anticipate a drop in the average to about eight hours. Subsequent babies average six to eight hours, but as labours vary considerably these times can only be a guide to you.

In order to pull up and open the cervix, the muscular uterus has to contract, producing contractions also known as 'labour pains'. In the last weeks of pregnancy, the uterus becomes thicker towards the top and thinner at the bottom. You may feel it tighten periodically at this time, as it makes preparatory (Braxton-Hicks) contractions. The tubular cervix is taken up by the uterus, until it is only an opening at the lower end. The plug of mucus, the 'show', which has sealed the cervix during pregnancy, then becomes loosened and falls out.

During labour the muscle fibres of your uterus contract, becoming shorter and fatter. However, when they relax between contractions they do not resume their original size but remain slightly smaller, so that the uterus gradually gets smaller with each contraction. Early contractions are often felt as low, intermittent backache, or period-type pain. Later, the feeling centres at the top of your 'bump', and more greatly resembles cramp. Contractions are also visible: the 'bump' becomes hard and appears to bulge forward. If you place your hand lightly upon it, you will feel this sensation heralding a contraction. How painful these contractions are is very subjective, but knowledge of their function, combined with conscious relaxation, can help you considerably. Every labour is individual, and it is unwise to assume that your labour will be the same as anyone else's, or even that it will run exactly the same course as a previous labour of your own.

The uterus continues to contract, each time opening the cervix wider. The contractions become more frequent, then more intense. At the height of labour, they may come every five minutes, lasting about two minutes, and followed by about three minutes' interval, that is, twelve per hour, with rest for thirty-six of the sixty minutes. This is a typical sequence, but the times may vary in each case.

As far as the baby is concerned, all this has the effect of living

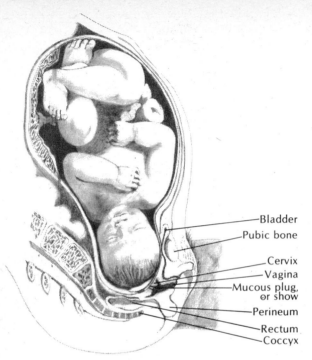

Bladder
Pubic bone
Cervix
Vagina
Mucous plug, or show
Perineum
Rectum
Coccyx

The baby in the uterus before labour

in a gradually deflating balloon, slowly but surely being directed towards the opening.

The bag of fluid protecting the baby helps to open the cervix by exerting firm, even pressure on it. At some point the pressure on the membraneous bag will become too great, and it will rupture, the warm fluid gushing or leaking forth, depending on how fully the baby's head is plugging the cervix. This process may be helped if the mother remains upright for as long as possible during labour.

These symptoms may happen in any order or combination:

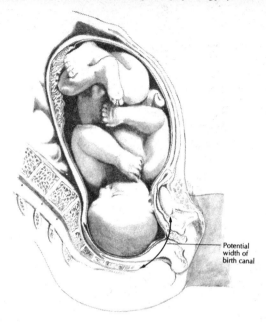

Potential
width of
birth canal

The waters about to break (the baby's head now rests inside the cervix)

Show   This is clear, white, pink, or brown mucus, sometimes streaked with blood, and about the size of a thimble. It is often flushed away when passing urine, and may not even be noticed. Alone, it is not an urgent sign and, unless accompanied by bright red bleeding, all that is necessary is to note when it happened and to check that all is prepared.

Contractions   Regular contractions of the uterus, continued over some time, are a definite sign of labour. At first they may only be weak and irregular, often stopping and restarting after a few hours. Unless you are specifically advised to the contrary, continue your usual activities steadily until the contractions are lasting for about three-quarters of a minute each, or are causing concern, at which time you should contact the midwife, and go to the place where your baby is to be born. A helpful guide as to when to leave for hospital is to know the time the journey will take (with adjustments for heavy traffic, fog, etc.) and consider how many contractions you could cope with in the car. This enables you to work out roughly the stage at which to leave home.

Waters breaking/ruptured membranes   This may happen as a first indication of labour, or it may not happen until later. Once the amniotic sac has ruptured and the cervix is dilated, there is a direct passage into the world for the baby and the midwife should be contacted. If the fluid is green, or there is heavy bleeding, you should ring for an ambulance to take you to hospital immediately as the baby may be distressed.

Transition to the second stage

There may be a transition phase at the end of the first stage of labour and before the second stage begins, when there is a change from contractions which open the cervix to those which push out the baby. This phase is often signalled by contractions which do not follow a pattern and which have increased intensity. It may be accompanied by nausea, vomiting, mental confusion, and a premature urge to bear down. The transition phase may last for one contraction or perhaps up to an hour, but it is not noticed in every labour.

The second stage

Once established, the second stage is one in which the labouring woman can work with her body, responding to the usually strong urge to bear down with each contraction. There is no longer any resistance from the cervix, and each contraction pushes the baby a fraction of the four inches along the birth canal. It may take one or two hours for a first baby, or perhaps only one or two contractions with subsequent ones. The birth canal is curved and good positioning is important to bring gravity to bear. If you are flat on your back, the baby will have to travel uphill for part of his journey. If you sit up, well-supported, or kneel—either leaning back on your heels or leaning forward and supported on a pillow resting on the bed-head —you can more easily help to push the baby towards birth. Some women find standing, supported by their labour companion, the most comfortable and the easiest way to give birth.

As the baby is manœuvred along with each push, the accordion-like folds of the vagina open out in front of his head, tucking themselves back into position as he passes on his way. Eventually he reaches the end of the birth canal and, with chin on chest, stretches the vaginal opening with the back of his

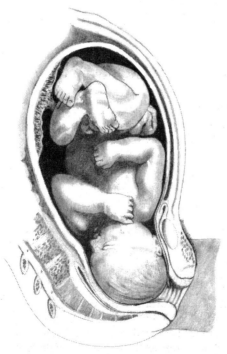

The baby in the birth canal

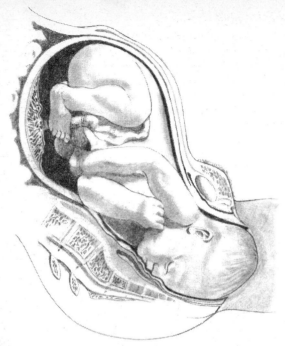

The baby's head about to be born

head, emerging as if through the neck of a tight pullover. At this point you are asked not to bear down, so that the baby is born without undue haste and avoiding possible damage to your perineal skin. Once his head is born, his shoulders twist round in the birth canal and his head turns sideways. The midwife checks that the umbilical cord is not hindering progress. One after the other his shoulders emerge, and his body slithers out. Thus he changes from expected baby to newborn in the welcome of your arms, sometimes protesting loudly, sometimes just viewing the world with a quizzical air.

The third stage

The final stage of labour is the delivery of the placenta. As the baby is being born, an injection is usually given to hasten the third stage, which may only take ten to fifteen minutes to complete. (This injection is a hormone, usually ergometrine (Syntometrine) and oxytocin, which helps the uterus to contract strongly. It has not been shown to be harmless to the baby or mother and it is thought possible that it delays the milk 'coming in' and could cause colic in the baby.) The physiological way to hasten the delivery of the placenta is to put the baby to

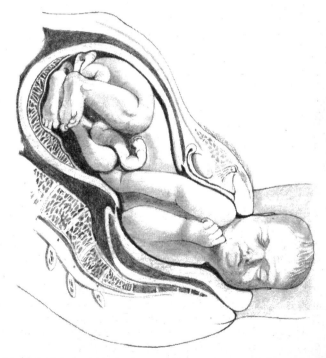

The birth of the head (the head rotates sideways after it emerges)

the breast: his suckling makes the uterus contract. The injection could always be given later if necessary. As your uterus decreases in volume, the area to which the placenta was clinging also decreases. When the baby no longer distends the uterus, it becomes much smaller, and the placenta is pushed off completely. The midwife notes external signs of this, and asks you to bear down with the next contraction, sometimes pulling gently on the cord, until the placenta arrives complete.

The contractions become irregular and subside. Although the placental site will continue to leak for several days, like menstruation, the uterus will have contracted sufficiently to prevent any excessive bleeding. During breastfeeding the contracting down of the uterus is stimulated and this decreases the

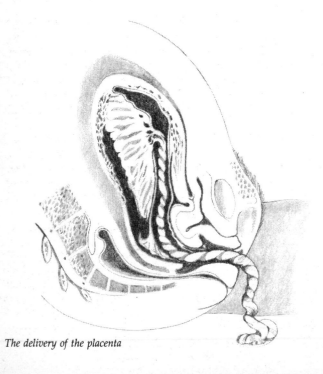

The delivery of the placenta

length of time of bleeding. You will probably feel the blood loss increasing during breastfeeding and you may pass clots of blood which otherwise would have stayed longer in the uterus. All this helps your uterus to return more quickly to a non-pregnant state.

The choice of birth at home

The NCT believes that women should be able to make an informed choice about where they have their babies, and that birth can be an enriching and happy experience either in hospital or at home.

In 1959 the Cranbrook Committee recommended that home confinements should be 30 per cent of the total, but by 1970 only 13 per cent of births in the United Kingdom took place at home, partly because of extra maternity provisions made to cope with what had been a rapidly expanding birth-rate a decade before. Now the birth-rate has declined dramatically, but the hospital beds remain and there is pressure to fill them lest they become uneconomic.

It is quite possible that you may feel ill at ease in hospital, especially if you have not had to stay in one previously. No matter how well intentioned everyone is, being in an alien atmosphere can have an inhibiting effect on your feelings of freedom to act as your instincts tell you, both during labour and in relating to your new baby. You will want to weigh this in the balance against other feelings of security which going to hospital may hold for you.

It is fair to say that there are good reasons for having a baby in hospital, as well as good reasons for maintaining a domiciliary service: the high quality of British midwifery has been justly acclaimed for many years.

Hospital care

There are two different kinds of hospital maternity care: GP units, including cottage hospitals and GP beds attached to or in consultant units, and consultant hospitals, which may have some GP beds in them, and where any mother who is ill or whose baby is at risk would be well advised to go.

Many women like GP units because they provide a homely atmosphere with a familiar doctor and midwife. If complications occur, the mother has to be moved to a consultant hospital, which should have a special care baby unit attached. If your doctor has already suggested a GP unit confinement, you can infer that you are 'low risk' and that it is safe to have your baby at home.

Good reasons for having a hospital birth

Toxaemia of pregnancy (pre-eclampsia).

A breech presentation For a home delivery to be relatively safe, the baby should be in a position with its head down before labour starts. With breech presentations the baby's bottom appears first, and the risks involved in delivery are greater.

A previous complicated birth Sometimes the complications experienced at one delivery will not necessarily be a reason for expecting problems next time. But a Caesarean section or a lot of bleeding after the previous birth are, for instance, reasons for having a subsequent hospital birth.

A premature birth This is one more than three weeks early, when the baby is likely to be small, and when an incubator and paediatric care should be available. For this reason it is wiser to have twins in hospital, as twins often come early.

Placenta praevia This is when the placenta is lying in the lower part of the uterus.

The statistics of perinatal mortality

Your doctor will be aware of perinatal mortality statistics, which indicate all babies who die in the first week of life (including actual stillbirths). In the last year for which detailed figures are available (1980) the perinatal mortality rate was 13.4 per 1,000 births in England and Wales (the stillbirth figure alone being

7.27 per 1,000). This is a noticeable improvement on the 1970 figures used for the first edition of this book, which were 23 per 1,000 (perinatal) and 13 per 1,000 (stillbirth).

The 'high risk' categories have also rearranged themselves since then, the highest risk now being to mothers over the age of 35 (18.4 per 1,000, the 'safest' age range now apparently being between 25 and 29); followed by the wives of unskilled workers (16.98 per 1,000 as against 9.7 per 1,000 for the wives of professional men); unsupported mothers (16.86 per 1,000 as against 12.83 per 1,000 for supported mothers); first babies (14 per 1,000 as against 10.4 per 1,000 for second babies); and babies whose mothers were born in the subcontinent of India (11.7 per 1,000 as against 7 per 1,000 for UK-born mothers).

Having said all that, it should be noted that even when the the risks are greatest, the vast majority of babies are born safely.

If you are thinking about a home birth you will want to know how they compare with hospital births for safety. Unfortunately it has become difficult to obtain helpful figures because the figure now quoted as the 'home birth' figure (very high at 25 per 1,000) no longer refers to births which have taken place at home by agreement; the figure includes all 'out of hospital' births—such as ambulance births and unplanned home births, concealed teenage pregnancies, etc. You may like to bear this in mind should anyone quote this figure to you.

Why home may be a good place

If the pregnancy is straightforward and the labour is likely to be normal, there are considerable advantages in having a baby at home. These include the practical advantages of avoiding travel to hospital when in labour, and being moved from room to room in hospital; avoiding unnecessary obstetric intervention; avoiding drugs which may adversely affect the baby; being able to keep mobile; and the relative ease in starting breastfeeding in one's own home and outside an institutional environment. There are the emotional benefits of feeling confident and relaxed in a familiar place; having continuity in maternity care; avoiding separation from other children in the family and allowing them to regard birth as a natural part of life; keeping mother and baby close together during the important minutes and hours after delivery; and feeling that you are retaining responsibility for your child's birth, with supportive rather than directive medical help.

The vital factor in preparing for a home confinement is to have the very best antenatal care possible.

How to set about getting a home confinement

The first person to talk to is your doctor, whom you may find understanding and helpful. Many doctors believe, however, that all babies should be born in hospital, and may therefore try to dissuade you from having a home birth—perhaps saying that you are risking the baby's life. (Birth can never be one hundred per cent safe, and of course some babies die wherever they are born. But this is something each couple will want to consider.)

It is a good idea for couples to discuss this together with the doctor, and to write down the advice you are given so that you can think about it coolly afterwards. You do not have to make a snap decision.

The doctor's professional responsibility means that he cannot make firm promises about home confinement early in pregnancy when it cannot yet be known if all will be well in five or six months' time. Most GPs who agree to a home confinement will only do so provided the pregnancy is straightforward. You should be prepared to make it clear to your doctor that you accept and understand this.

The general practitioner obstetrician to whom you go for maternity care need not be your usual GP and you can ask to have maternity care from another GP. Often only one partner in a practice does maternity work anyway. If you are thinking of a home confinement it is worth asking the GP as soon as pregnancy is diagnosed if his or her partner is prepared to do home deliveries provided everything is likely to be straight-forward, and if not whether you can have the name of a GP obstetrician who is.

Should your own doctor not know of a GP who does home

confinements, you may wish to contact the Area Nursing Officer (at your Area Health Authority office) asking for the names of GPs on the obstetric list who sometimes do home confinements. You will probably be put in touch also with the Community Nursing Officer, who supervises the community midwives. Let her know you feel strongly about a home confinement and ask how midwifery cover can be arranged.

If you come to a dead end, write explaining what has happened to your Community Health Council, and ask if they can help. You may like to send copies of your letter to the Area Nursing Officer and to the Family Practitioner Committee, whose address you can get from your Area Health Authority office.

According to her conditions of service, established by the Central Midwives' Board, a midwife called when you are in labour at home must attend.

If you already have a GP obstetrician who is opposed to home confinements or if you are attending a consultant unit but want to have a home confinement instead, it is probably best to put your reasons for wanting a home birth in writing to the doctor concerned and to the Area Nursing Officer. Try to be very clear and unemotional about it. It is important that your partner agrees, and a good idea to sign the letter jointly. If your reason for wanting a home confinement is to avoid going to a particular hospital, explain why in detail.

Once a home birth has been agreed, the midwife will look at your home to advise you how to make everything ready. The place should be clean and convenient, with running water, but there is no need to try to reproduce hospital conditions.

As the estimated date approaches, the midwife will leave a sterile maternity pack in your home, and give you any necessary instructions. You will need to provide a bucket and a few bowls and things. There is usually no need to rearrange the bedroom, though it is easier if the bed is at right angles to the wall and can be approached from three sides.

When labour starts When you feel that your labour is

established, contact the midwife. She may ask you to let her know, before she goes out on her rounds in the morning, if you think the baby is likely to be born that day.

Home helps   Social services departments may be able to provide home helps after home confinements for a period of 14 days—or longer if the GP considers it is necessary. You will have to contribute a certain proportion towards her pay. Your husband may also wish to take a week or more off work.

Sources of further information   You may like to talk to someone who has had a home birth in your area. Other people who may be able to help are: your NCT teacher; The Society to Support Home Confinements, Margaret Whyte, 17 Laburnum Avenue, Durham City; The Patients' Association, Suffolk House, Banbury Road, Oxford; The Association for Improvement in Maternity Services (AIMS), Beverley Beach, 21 Iver Lane, Iver, Bucks. SL0 9LH; The Association of Radical Midwives (ARM), c/o 8A The Drive, Wimbledon, London SW20; Birmingham Birth Centre, c/o Phyl Doneghan, 18 Mackenzie Road, Moseley, Birmingham B11 4EL.

Remember . . .   if you plan to have a baby at home it is vitally important to have good antenatal care as well as leading a healthy life during pregnancy. See your doctor regularly and take his advice. Do not take any medicine or tablets without consulting your GP even when you are not absolutely sure you are pregnant (it is in early pregnancy that the worst damage can be done to the fetus). Avoid eating synthetic foods and if you smoke give up if you possibly can, because nicotine reduces the amount of oxygen that reaches the baby. Go to antenatal classes and learn all you can about helping yourself in labour.

A guide to labour for expectant parents

The following is an outline of a normal labour. Each labour is highly individual and no exact pattern can be guaranteed. Do not expect a set series of events but be prepared to accept whatever your particular labour brings. Enjoy knowing what to do to help yourself as much as you are able. Set yourself no other aims.

In this guide, each phase of labour is set out in distinct parts: 'What is happening', 'Helping yourself', 'Relaxation/breathing/ position', and 'Partner's help'. This is done for easy reference and to tie together the subjects we have mentioned separately in previous sections.

Prelude to labour

What is happening   You may notice some of the following: lightening (when the baby's head drops into the pelvis) two to four weeks before a first baby, perhaps just before labour with subsequent babies; frequent 'practice' contractions, felt as a hardening of the abdomen; increased vaginal mucus discharge; slight weight loss a few days before labour begins; less activity in the baby; a spurt of energy in you, the mother, one or two days before labour; wind in the bowel and, sometimes, frequent and loose motions; pelvic pressure. The 'show' may be now or at the onset of labour: a plug of mucus with perhaps a streak of blood. You may lose this gradually over a period of days.

Helping yourself   Don't overdo things; simplify housework. From the time you are eight months pregnant have your hospital suitcase packed or, for a home confinement, have your maternity pack and personal requirements handy where you plan to have the delivery and have the baby clothes, cot blankets, and sheets aired. Protect your mattress in case your waters leak at the onset of labour. Don't concentrate too hard on the expected date of confinement, which is after all only a guide.

Relaxation/breathing Use calm breathing to help you relax. This will help you to conserve energy and overcome sleeplessness. Remember to keep practising the pelvic floor exercises, and make good use of massage techniques for better relaxation.

Partner's help Warn the appropriate people at work that you're intending to take time off in the near future. Make sure your partner always knows where to contact you. Offer diversions —make some dates for after the baby is due. Know all the necessary telephone numbers, the route to the hospital, and the parking places there. Keep your petrol topped up. Massage is relaxing for both of you.

Spontaneous labour—onset

What is happening You may notice one, or any combination, of the following: regular contractions, felt as low abdominal discomfort, backache, period-type pain, or similar; the 'show'; breaking or leaking of the waters.

Helping yourself Check the signs; time the contractions occasionally, and report to the hospital or midwife as advised. If the 'show' is very heavy and includes blood, report it at once. If the waters break, with or without contractions, also report this at once. Food will provide you with energy, but taken now it must be easily digestible, so avoid roughage, milk, soft bread, fats, and acid foods. Select from tea, plain biscuits, clear broth/ beef extract drink, lightly boiled/poached egg, thin slice of crisp white toast.

Relaxation/breathing Use this phase to relax fully, with calm, easy breathing through a relaxed mouth. Keep in touch with what your body is doing. Visualize the cervix just beginning to open.

Partner's help Check final preparations—lists may help. Maintain as calm and unhurried an atmosphere as possible. Suggest light activities to avoid a boring wait. Make sandwiches to take to hospital for your own use. Perhaps prepare a light meal.

Early first stage

What is happening The cervix is being drawn up by the power-ful muscles at the top of the uterus, and it is beginning to dilate.

Helping yourself In daytime, continue light activity; at night, rest, or if very excited get up and have a drink (tea, beef extract drink) and then relax in a comfortable position, or take a hot-water bottle back to bed. A warm bath is nice, if the waters haven't ruptured, or a shower if they have.

Relaxation/breathing Use calm rhythmic breathing to help you relax.

Partner's help Help her to remain cheerful by chatting between contractions. Wear cool clothes for hospital and avoid nylon shirts.

As the first stage progresses . . .

What is happening The contractions become stronger and perhaps closer together. They may last longer too. The midwife may see you and ask about progress so far. You may still be carrying on normally at home if labour doesn't seem very advanced to you. When you do go to hospital, or the midwife arrives at home, you will be examined internally and perhaps offered an enema (liquid injected into the bowel) or suppository (substance introduced into the rectum) in order to assist you to empty your bowels. You can decline these if you prefer. As the contractions get stronger, the cervix will dilate more rapidly. You will find the need for positive support from those around you and won't want to be distracted from the job in hand.

Helping yourself Once you are having strong regular contrac-tions and labour is established you may not feel like eating, but if you do, restrict yourself to tea, rose-hip syrup, plain biscuits, thin crisp white toast (preferably without butter). You may enjoy a glucose tablet, but as they all contain a trace of acid restrict this to occasional use. Being up and about is likely to feel better and help this stage pass more quickly, but be guided in this by your own preferences. Be prepared for a more painful contraction after an examination or enema. Ask the midwife not to examine you during a contraction unless there is a good reason for doing so (it can give a better estimate of dilatation). Remember to empty your bladder from time to time, as you may not be aware of its being full. A full bladder can slow down the descent of the baby's head. Ask someone to rub your back if you have a 'back labour'. Try to visualize the cervix opening, not necessarily as it is, but as an appealing image, such as a bud opening into a flower.

Relaxation/breathing/position   An upright position is more efficient and less painful for most people. Relax during the journey to hospital and continue to give priority to full relaxation. If in bed, find a comfortable position with plenty of pillows. Try experimenting with all kinds of positions (for example for a backache labour try positions which relieve pressure: on all fours, or sitting astride a chair leaning your arms forwards on to the chair back). Breathe as seems comfortable and relax as contractions become stronger. Don't resist the good work your uterus is doing.

Partner's help   In hospital, remind the midwife of any specific requests you have. Remind your partner to relax and help with changes of position, supporting her if necessary. Make sure she is as upright as possible. Lying flat can cause distress to the baby. Explain to the staff about the breathing if they interrupt during a contraction. Remind your partner to empty her bladder—every two hours at least. Support her in any decisions about pain relief and insist on an examination first.

Late first stage

What is happening   Dilatation continues, usually at a quicker pace, as contractions become more frequent and stronger. The waters may break now or later. It is usually better not to have them ruptured artificially.

Helping yourself   Try not to think of anything but the present moment. Just respond to the contraction you're having now. Remember that contractions only come one at a time. Visualize the cervix half open now, with the baby waiting to come through. Rocking during contractions can be very soothing.

Relaxation/breathing/position   Breathe as you find comfortable to help relaxation. Finish each contraction with a deeper breath and a smile. Relax with this 'resting' breath. Change position from time to time—try kneeling, or supporting yourself on knees and elbows, or lying on your left side well propped up with pillows. (See illustrations on pp. 57, 61, 62.) If you over-breathe (hyperventilate) and feel dizzy, or have tingly fingers, breathe in and out into your hands cupped round your mouth and nose, then breathe more gently. You may want to use distraction techniques: a song, poem, counting in threes, or just mouthing 'hout' on every breath.

Partner's help   Your partner may not want to talk much. Help her to stay in the present (see 'Helping yourself'). Try massage if she likes to be touched. Give her sips of water and sponge her face if she is uncomfortably hot. Join in distraction techniques and keep up eye contact. Help with changes of position.

Transition from first to second stage

What is happening   You may now be moved to the delivery room. There may be strong irregular contractions, close together, making you feel muddled. There might be an urge to bear down in the middle of a contraction, before the cervix is fully dilated. If you are told you have an 'anterior lip' it means that part of the cervix has not been fully pulled up and may be damaged if you push too soon. The contractions may become overwhelming as the cervix is now very stretched. This can produce panic and loss of rhythm. You may feel irritable, angry, weepy, hot, or cold; you may shake, or vomit.

Helping yourself   Tell yourself this is the climax of the first stage and the baby will soon be here. Make noises if you feel like it. Soon you will be able to push and it will be far less painful. Perhaps use Entonox—it is now too late for pethidine. Ask for an examination before beginning to push strongly.

Relaxation/breathing/position   If you feel like pushing too early, blow out to counteract this urge. Take four shallow breaths, with a sharp blow out on the fourth. Perhaps say to yourself 'I will not push'—one breath on each word. You may like to do this into cupped hands, so you can hear your breathing and avoid hyperventilating. If contractions should stop (for instance due to a change of room) relax, enjoy the rest, and wait for them to come back. Upright positions help with dilatation, or try the knees/elbows position for extra comfort (kneel on a firm surface, lean forward on to your forearms, and rest your head on your arms).

Partner's help Reassure your partner and remind her that she's nearly there. Accept and understand tears or tantrums. Don't argue. Encourage transition breathing and help with position; perhaps suggest knees and elbows for an anterior lip (see 'What is happening'), or kneeling upright. She may feel out of contact or even frightened at this point. Don't leave her alone.

Second stage

What is happening Contractions during this stage may be several minutes apart. The cervix is fully dilated, as your baby moves down the vagina. Soon the head can be seen. The pressure of the head has variously been described as feeling like a huge bowel movement or a large ripe grapefruit. There is a very strong bearing-down urge and a great sense of bulging and stretching. In some rare instances this bearing-down urge may be absent. As your baby's head slides out into the world there may be a burning sensation, followed by a feeling of numbness.

Helping yourself Go with the contractions, and remember to relax your pelvic floor. The midwife will guide you during the delivery. You may like to lift your baby out yourself and hold him close. When asked not to push, lift your head and pant, with mouth, pelvic floor, and legs all relaxed.

Relaxation/breathing/position Try to be aware of how the waves of pushing during contractions happen naturally, with your breathing adapting accordingly. If your mouth is relaxed, your vagina will be too. Let gravity help by staying as upright as you can. Kneeling is good, as is supported squatting during a contraction. You may find that you wish to hold your breath for short periods whilst you push, or you may find that blowing out steadily can be helpful. If all is going well the uterus can do most of the work on its own. This is more likely if you are upright. Don't hold your breath for long spells. Push as your uterus seems to dictate.

Partner's help Do all you can to ensure that your partner is in the position which suits her best. Explain to the staff what you wish to do. For a supported semi-squat, stand close behind her, supporting her under her arms with your fingers linked tightly across her upper chest and using your whole body for support. Take her whole weight during the contraction. If she wants to watch the actual delivery, someone could hold a mirror. Sensations and emotions at this point are very intense and it is exciting and perhaps even rather disturbing to know that your baby will soon be here.

Third stage

What is happening As the baby is born, an injection of Syntometrine is often given routinely in order to prevent post-partum haemorrhage and to help expel the placenta. If you wish to do without Syntometrine unless there is good reason for it in your particular case, you will need to have queried this in advance. At the time it will be over before you're aware of it. Putting your baby to your breast, or simply having skin contact, may help to expel the placenta naturally. It is expelled with another pushing contraction. You will be washed and made comfortable, possibly whilst still holding the baby. You will probably be offered a cup of tea. Stitching up is done if necessary.

Helping yourself Push to deliver the placenta when the midwife asks you to. Enjoy a peaceful time getting to know your new baby, who will have all faculties alert to get to know both parents.

Relaxation/breathing/position Remember gravity can still help with the delivery of the placenta. Relax if being stitched and whilst giving your baby a first breastfeed. Be careful about positioning the baby when breastfeeding so that your nipple is not being pulled.

Partner's help   Support your partner in any decisions you have made about treatment at this stage. Take time to get to know your new child—he needs your love and protection now.

Postnatal period

What is happening   There may be after-pains, especially during breastfeeds. They indicate that the uterus is being made to contract back to its original size. Bleeding (lochia) may continue for two weeks or more and increase after excessive activity. Take this as a warning to slow down.

Helping yourself   Welcome the contractions causing after-pains, if necessary using your relaxation techniques again. Smiling helps to relax you. Don't rush to get back to your old routine and don't expect too much of yourself in the first few weeks.

Relaxation   Relax during every breastfeed and always take care to make yourself comfortable, positioning your baby close to your nipple.

Partner's help   Try to take every opportunity to handle and care for your baby, even in hospital, so that you feel less at a disadvantage at the home-coming.

A guide to medical procedures during labour

Admission procedures

Much modern maternity care has become routine and procedures remain after they have been shown to be unnecessary.

Even now in some hospitals every woman has her pubic and vulval hair shaved off, is given an enema, and is told to take a bath or shower. None of these procedures is essential. If you wish to avoid any or all of this ritual, you would be well advised to discuss the admission procedure with those who will care for you, before your labour begins. However, although inessential, you may find a bath or shower pleasurable. The warmth of the water may stimulate your contractions and, if you can make yourself comfortable in the bath, you may find it easier to relax during contractions.

Management of the first stage of labour

Companionship   Most maternity hospitals now allow fathers, or other labour companions, to be present throughout labour. Preferably this should be discussed and settled with the hospital antenatally. It should give you continuous support so that you never feel alone. But, in some places, partners are still asked to leave if any procedure, however minor, is carried out, such as giving an injection or making a vaginal examination. If you want your partner to stay, ask the doctor whether it would be possible. Not infrequently, a nurse or midwife will ask a partner to leave before the doctor comes, on the assumption that the doctor will prefer it that way, whereas the doctor may be happy to allow a partner to stay. Make it clear that your partner wants to stay to help you, not to interfere with medical procedures.

Your companion may be asked to put on a hospital gown and to wear a cap and mask.

Food and fluid   It is usual practice in most maternity hospitals to forbid taking food and fluid by mouth during labour, in case you have to have a general anaesthetic at some stage, when you might bring back and inhale what is in your stomach. This is not an unreasonable precaution, especially as you may not feel like eating or drinking very much, and as your stomach empties and digests more slowly in labour. However, your mouth may feel dry and to moisten it is a welcome relief that should not be denied. You may like to have a light meal at home in the early stages of labour and to have some cracked ice to suck later on in labour. Orange or lemon juice added to the water before freezing makes the ice especially refreshing. In some places you will be given a white chalky mixture (magnesium trisilicate) to drink every few hours during your labour to make the contents of your stomach less acid, and less likely to damage your lungs should you be given a general anaesthetic and inhale any stomach contents.

Intravenous fluids   Some doctors like women in labour to have a 'drip' of fluid through a needle into a vein (intravenous infusion), because the energy that you use during labour demands a constant supply of fluid. This is not necessary in normal labour.

Vaginal examinations   Progress in labour is judged by noting how often your contractions are coming, and how strong and how long they are. More exactly, progress is assessed by measuring how wide open the cervix is and by noting the way in which the baby's presenting part (the leading bit of the baby, usually the top of the head, or vertex, and rarely the bottom, or breech) descends through the birth canal on internal examination. The opening of the cervix is measured in centimetres (1–10), or occasionally in 1–5 finger-breadths. When the cervix is fully open (dilated to 10 cm) the second stage of labour is said to begin. In some hospitals, it is routine practice to assess dilatation of the cervix by vaginal examination repeated every two to four hours. When the waters break it is usual to make a vaginal examination to make sure that a loop of the baby's umbilical cord has not slipped below the head where it could be compressed against the cervix. It is also advisable to make sure that the baby is unlikely to arrive within the next three hours by checking the dilatation of the cervix before pain-relieving drugs are given or repeated.

Emptying your bladder   Late in labour, because the bladder is pulled upwards as your cervix opens and the baby's head goes down the birth canal, you may find it difficult to urinate or have no desire to empty your bladder. This is especially true under epidural analgesia. The midwives will keep an eye on this, and if necessary pass a tube (catheter) into your bladder to empty it. Keeping the bladder empty gives more room for the baby's head.

Analgesia Most midwives and doctors expect you to require pain relief during labour. There is much emphasis in our society on avoiding any sensation which cannot be guaranteed pleasant and painless. One doctor even went so far as to say that women wanting to experience natural childbirth must have some sort of mental derangement and feel a need to be punished.

In the first place discomfort and pain are differently tolerated by different people so that the decision about when you require relief must logically be your own decision. Without suggesting that there is any merit in suffering for suffering's sake, we believe that many mothers would rather suffer some discomfort or pain than risk affecting their baby by consuming drugs, and some will accept a certain amount of pain in order to experience also the sensations of giving birth. However, there are too many unknown quantities about a labour which has not started for it to be wise for you to take up beforehand a rigid position in relation to drugs, but always ask the staff about the effects on you and your baby of any drugs which might be offered.

If you are admitted at night in early labour, often you will be offered a sleeping tablet. If you are unaccustomed to taking them, this is probably an unwise time to experiment because you will need your wits about you to cope with progressive contractions. Later on the drug most often used is pethidine in a dose of 100 or 150 mg (NB: some mothers have found only a quarter of this amount sufficient to be helpful) given by injection. Often pethidine is combined with a tranquillizer or antihistamine, which may help to counteract nausea and vomiting, but which also increases drowsiness and gives a feeling of detachment. Some women find this frightening and hate the sensation of knowing they could do something to help themselves but that the drug has taken away their ability to communicate or to concentrate long enough to move. Injections of pain-relieving drugs should seldom be repeated more than every four hours. Later on in labour it is wise to find out the progress you have made before having injections, since if the birth of your baby can be expected within three hours the drugs given may delay the onset of his breathing. There is an antidote which can be given to the baby if necessary.

As birth comes nearer, instead of pain-relieving injections you may breathe a mixture of gas (nitrous oxide) and oxygen—Entonox—during contractions in order to help relieve the pain. This inhaled analgesia should be used right at the beginning of each contraction and only about four or five breaths should be taken so that you are alert to use it at the start of the next contraction.

Many women find that they can handle their labours without taking any form of drugs, but just using relaxation and breathing techniques. However, labour should never be a mere endurance test, and if you feel in need of extra relief you should not hesitate to ask for it. Since pethidine is a mood-enhancing drug it is best to request it before you become distressed. The time to ask is when you begin to feel that you cannot cope *between contractions*. Pethidine is a poor analgesic (i.e. it won't take away pain), but it can help you to relax and sleep between contractions. Be sure, however, to ask for an examination to find out the dilatation of your cervix as you may be reaching the end of the first stage, in which case the drug would not take effect before you wanted to start to push your baby out in the second stage of labour. Pethidine is known to depress the baby's sucking reflex, so if your baby is sleepy and slow to suck at first, do not worry. The effect of the drug will wear off, and feeding will become much easier.

Epidural analgesia   The nerves which conduct sensations from the uterus, cervix, and vagina to the brain leave the lower spinal cord, which is surrounded by your backbone (vertebral column). The nerves can be temporarily blocked so that they no longer conduct impulses by exposing them to a solution of local anaesthetic. In epidural anaesthesia this is done by placing a thin plastic tube between two of your lower vertebrae into the spinal canal just outside the spinal cord and near the nerve roots to your lower body and legs. The tube is threaded through a needle, inserted after first numbing your back. Once the plastic tube is in place, the needle is withdrawn and the local anaesthetic solution is injected. You will then feel numb in the lower half of your body and legs. You may still be aware that your uterus is contracting, but you will not feel it as pain. The effect of an epidural varies with the placement of the tube and the dose of anaesthetic used, and usually lasts between one and three hours. When one dose wears off, further doses of the anaesthetic solution can be given through the plastic tube, which is left in place until your baby has been born.

The advantages of epidural analgesia are that you remain fully awake and free from pain without the need for other pain-relieving and sedative drugs. Because epidural analgesia causes a drop in blood pressure, it is useful for women whose blood pressure is high. Epidural analgesia can also be used instead of putting you to sleep with a general anaesthetic to carry out forceps, breech, and twin delivery as well as Caesarean section.

The disadvantages of epidural analgesia are that your movement is restricted, it requires careful supervision, and there is an increased need to use forceps for delivery. It may be effective on only one side of your body. Many women with epidurals find it difficult to push their babies out themselves, because they have lost their pelvic floor sensations. However, you can be helped to push out your baby yourself, if you are guided when to push with your contractions. Epidural analgesia requires special skill and experience, and may not be available at all times, or even at all in some maternity hospitals. Some women suffer severe headache or backache after an epidural and some have difficulty in passing urine. Your baby may have feeding problems after birth.

A recent survey has shown that women given an epidural were far less satisfied with their labour in retrospect than those who did not have an epidural. Midwives have noticed that many women who have had an epidural do not seem to experience the joy and exhilaration usual after a natural labour.

Women's bodies are designed to give birth to babies and there is a complicated mechanism which starts this process and maintains its progress: a mechanism both psychological and physical which begins in pregnancy and continues into motherhood.

Monitoring the health of your baby   When the waters break, the fluid should be clear, straw-coloured, or milky. Sometimes it contains white greasy flecks—the vernix, which is a protective secretion from the glands of the baby's skin. All this is perfectly normal. If, however, the water that drains out is stained green or dark yellow from the meconium in the baby's bowel, this is a warning that the baby may be short of oxygen and the midwife or doctor will want to make sure that the baby is born soon.

Normally the baby's heart beats at a rate of between 120 and 160 per minute, the actual speed at any moment varying quite considerably between these limits. The heart-rate can be counted by listening to it through a stethoscope or with ultrasound (Sonicaid). During normal labour the baby's heart-rate, your pulse and blood pressure are recorded at first every hour, later every half-hour, and towards the end of labour perhaps after every contraction. Warning of danger can be provided if the fetal heart-rate is recorded and observed continuously. This is called monitoring and can be done automatically after picking up the heartbeat from sound or ultrasound waves, or from electrical signals. Usually a receiver for the signals from the baby's heart is strapped to your abdomen, which also records the contractions of your uterus by means of a pressure-sensitive gauge. A cable connects the receiver to a computer which calculates the heart-rate and provides a continuous written record of what is happening. Some obstetricians prefer to record the baby's heart-rate directly by attaching a metal clip to the baby's head through the vagina and cervix after the membranes have ruptured.

Some hospitals follow a policy of monitoring every woman continuously throughout labour. They do this because they believe that it is in the best interests of the baby, but it has the disadvantage that you are unable to get out of bed and it is difficult even in bed to move around freely. You can ask to be monitored sitting in a comfortable armchair. It can be argued whether or not real advantage is to be gained by continuous monitoring of every labour, rather than by selecting only those women who have signs of early fetal distress or in whom there is some reason to suspect that the baby may become distressed, for example, women with raised blood pressure, those who have had difficulties in earlier pregnancies, or those who are ten days or more past the expected date of delivery. Some hospitals have more recently developed 'telemetric' monitoring equipment which allows the mother to walk around, so that at least the frustrations and discomforts of being restrained in bed are removed and therefore some of the negative aspects of monitoring. It has been suggested that many of the problems recorded by the monitors used on mothers in bed are actually caused by her being in a recumbent position.

Acceleration of labour   Labour lasting more than 24 hours is not generally good, either for you or your baby. If uterine contractions are weak, infrequent and/or irregular, they can be made more effective in dilating the cervix by a variety of means:

If you have been lying or semi-reclining in bed, changing your position to a more upright one or walking around will enable gravity to draw the baby's head down on to the cervix, strengthen the contractions, and speed the dilatation.

If the contractions are weak because you have had a long tiring labour, eating something or having a glucose drip can help.

Kneeling or reclining and relaxing in a comfortably hot bath can also stimulate the contractions.

Failing these suggestions, dripping the hormone oxytocin (Syntocinon) into a vein at a carefully measured rate will accelerate the labour.

Many obstetricians believe that more than 12 hours in labour is undesirable, and will, therefore, accelerate labour sooner than other doctors who are willing for labour to last a little longer. The rate of progress in labour generally speeds up after the membranes rupture. The membranes can be ruptured artificially for this purpose by nicking a hole in them as they bulge through the opening cervix with a pair of forceps guided along the fingers during a vaginal examination.

The second stage of labour

You may feel that the second stage is the really positive part of your labour, when you can work with your body to bring your baby into the world. You may value your partner's support and companionship particularly now and want to share with him the moving experience of the delivery itself.

An episiotomy   This is a cut made in the skin and muscles to enlarge the opening to the vagina so that the baby's head can pass out more easily and/or more quickly. An episiotomy should not usually be made without first numbing the tissues that are to be cut by injecting a local anaesthetic solution. Many obstetricians encourage the almost routine use of episiotomy, especially in women having their first babies, although other obstetricians maintain that this is not necessary. Episiotomies *are* necessary if they are needed to protect you and your baby from injury, for example, if the baby is born too early (before 34 weeks), if the delivery is complicated and instruments are used, if you are too tired from your efforts so far, or if the baby is in distress and the birth is imminent.

Without an episiotomy many women will suffer tears in the skin and the superficial muscles guarding the entrance to the vagina, but episiotomies are often more extensive than required, and tears are often less painful and heal more quickly than episiotomies. Furthermore, an episiotomy may deprive you of the internal sensations that help you to push your baby out. (For more details about coping with an episiotomy, see p. 150.)

Cutting the cord Some obstetricians advocate that the cord should be allowed to stop pulsating before it is cut, to give the baby as much oxygenated blood as possible, but it is still common for the umbilical cord to be cut very soon after the baby is born. Then the midwife usually sucks the baby's nose and mouth clear of mucus and fluid.

The third stage of labour

To cut down the amount of blood that is lost when the placenta separates, it is usual to give you an injection of a mixture of ergometrine and oxytocin (Syntometrine) just as the baby is about to be born. The placenta should then separate with the birth of the baby so that it follows the baby's bottom to rest in the cervix and upper vagina, and can then be delivered almost immediately. This is most often done by the method of cord traction and supra-pubic pressure: which means that the midwife takes the cord in one hand and with the other presses on the abdomen to steady the uterus. By pulling the cord down she draws the placenta out of the vagina. If nature is left to herself, you can push the placenta out yourself. Suckling the baby at the breast also causes the uterus to contract and to expel the placenta. It has been suggested that Syntometrine delays breast milk 'coming in': certainly it has not been proved to be without side-effects.

A guide to obstetric interventions

Should any of the following be proposed to you, or become necessary, here is an outline of what you may expect to happen and how to cope in the circumstances.

Induction of labour

Occasionally this is advisable for medical reasons. You should be given a full explanation and time to discuss the situation with your partner, if you wish to, before the procedure is started.

What is happening A prostaglandin pessary will probably be inserted to begin with. Later the membranes may be ruptured. If this is not effective a hormone drip will be set up. This feeds oxytocin into your blood and labour usually starts within the next hour or two. A pessary alone may take longer to work. You are likely to be attached to an external monitor which works by ultrasound. This monitors your contractions and your baby's heartbeat on a machine beside the bed. When you are induced contractions are likely to start off more strongly than otherwise and the labour may be quicker, though not all are.

Helping yourself If you are attached to a drip then movement is restricted, so try to get comfortable to start with, perhaps asking to sit in a comfortable chair, instead of being in bed. If the contractions are running into each other, ask the midwife to adjust the drip. The drip will not be removed until a few hours after your baby is born. Move often and whenever you are uncomfortable: ask the staff to help you. Remind companions not to become too centred on the monitoring machine—you are still the expert on your own sensations. Be prepared to use breathing and relaxation right from the start.

Relaxation/breathing Relax as fully as you can, breathing in the way you find most helpful. If the contractions are difficult, use lighter and slightly faster breathing. Try visualizing the cervix stretching open slowly and gently, to counteract any undue panic caused by the stronger contractions resulting from induction. Think positively: your baby will soon be born!

Partner's help Try to be with your partner from the beginning of the induction procedure. Support her through eye contact and breathe with her as contractions become stronger. Help her to relax and try to stay relaxed yourself. Don't forget to use massage.

Continuous electronic monitoring (external monitoring)

This is sometimes suggested in a normal labour.

What is happening An ultrasonic transducer is attached to your abdomen by a belt of some kind in order to monitor your baby's heartbeat and your contractions—both of which can be detected by simpler means. The trappings can be uncomfortable and restricting. If no unusual readings are found within thirty minutes or so, you can request the removal of the equipment. A portable ('telemetric') system may be used which would allow you to walk about.

Helping yourself   Query the need for the monitoring. Remember that your baby is receiving continuous ultrasonic waves while the equipment is in use. Remind attendants that you know better than a machine how you are feeling. Stay as upright as possible with plenty of pillows for support.

Relaxation/position   Try to get comfortable. If the belt keeps slipping off, it won't be giving accurate readings and the midwife will need to readjust it. Focus on your own sensations. If you like, you can use the machine as an indicator of when a contraction is starting.

Partner's help   Support your partner in any request for the belt to be removed after a spell of normal readings. Don't watch the machine all the time—it's not having the baby.

Fetal scalp monitor (internal monitoring)

This gives a continuous indication of the baby's ability to respond to the stresses of labour.

What is happening   An electrode is attached to your baby's scalp, either by a hook or a small screw, in order to monitor your baby's heartbeat. The membranes must be ruptured before a scalp monitor is attached. At the same time a catheter in the uterus is used to measure your contractions. This is restricting for you and can, in itself, affect the baby's heartbeat. The same information may possibly be obtained by external monitoring, but internal monitoring can be much more accurate. Your baby may develop an infected spot on his head later.

Helping yourself   Query the need for this. If you do agree to it, realize that your baby may need especially sensitive care afterwards as consolation and reassurance. If the labour is progressing normally, ask for short spells of external monitoring instead.

Relaxation/breathing   This may make relaxing and breathing calmly more difficult. Try to remain positive and keep your attention on your immediate feelings in spite of all the machines.

Partner's help   Support any decisions about monitoring and explain your wishes to the staff. Elicit explanations from them about reasons for suggesting a monitor. You need not agree to routine practices for which there is no medical indication.

Fetal blood sampling

What is happening   A sample of your baby's blood is taken at intervals from the scalp in order to test the pH (acidity) level of the blood and thus detect any oxygen deprivation. Often very unpleasant for the baby, who may develop an infected spot as a result. Only some hospitals use this method.

Helping yourself   Query the need for this. If you agree to it, console your baby after the birth.

Relaxation/position   Your legs will be in stirrups for the few minutes this takes. The test might be repeated later.

Partner's help   Be certain that this is called for before agreeing to it. Help with making your partner comfortable.

Acceleration of labour

What is happening   The same hormone drip as is used for an induction may be used to speed up a slow labour. Contractions may suddenly become longer and stronger. An enema may achieve the same effect. A soak in a hot bath is also very effective in stimulating contractions.

Helping yourself   Try to avoid the necessity for this by keeping up and about and not going into hospital too soon (unless, of course, there is some specific reason for doing so).

Relaxation/breathing   Lighter, slightly faster breathing for stronger contractions. Perhaps a distraction technique, or massage, too.

Partner's help Help to deal with each contraction as it comes. If contractions suddenly become stronger a lot of support will be required.

Artificial rupture of the membranes

What is happening Forceps are used to make a hole in the membranes as they bulge through the cervix. This is sometimes uncomfortable or even painful and the following contractions may be stronger as a result of the procedure. The baby should be delivered within twenty-four hours because of the risk of infection.

Helping yourself Query the need for this. You may not wish your labour to be hurried on in this way, or for your baby's head to be pressed directly against the cervix, causing swelling of the scalp.

Relaxation/breathing Relax while it is being done and be prepared for the need for lighter breathing for the next contraction.

Partner's help You may be asked to leave the room for this. It only takes a few minutes. Come back soon. Be ready for labour to accelerate afterwards.

Episiotomy

What is happening A surgical incision is made to widen the birth outlet. In a normal labour, an upright position and relaxed pelvic floor reduce the likelihood of this being needed. For forceps it is almost always essential.

Helping yourself Ask to deliver in an upright position. Allow the second stage to proceed in its own time, without hurry. If you do have an episiotomy insist on a local anaesthetic for the stitches and possibly use Entonox as well.

Relaxation Try to relax.

Partner's help You don't have to watch, but you may neverthe-less hear the sound of the cut being made.

See also p. 150.

Forceps delivery (or Ventouse delivery)

This may be needed for the following reasons: failure of the baby to progress in spite of strong pushes; protection of a very small baby; a breech birth, where delivery of the head needs to be slow and controlled; distress in the baby or mother.

What is happening Forceps are used by the doctor who places them on either side of your baby's head, where his hands cannot reach, in order to aid the delivery of your baby's head.

Helping yourself Note that some consultants go purely by time in the second stage and that if your baby is not distressed there is no urgency. For a small baby or a breech birth, Entonox sometimes helps to control a delivery which is too fast, and also relieves the discomfort of the forceps delivery.

Relaxation/breathing/position In the case of failure to progress, adopt an upright position—kneeling or supported squat. This may make forceps unnecessary. Should they be necessary, relax as much as possible and push when the doctor pulls.

Partner's help Help your partner to change position and to find the best one. You may be asked to leave. Come in again as soon as you hear the baby cry. If you are present, your role is to be as supportive and reassuring as you can through what may be an unpleasant few minutes. Stay at the 'head end' of the bed.

Analgesics

The best pain relief in labour is relaxation combined with the caring encouragement and support of a known partner and a midwife. For most labours this is all that is needed, but there are many reasons why you might require more.

Entonox (nitrous oxide and oxygen)

This has no long-term effects on the baby.

What is happening You breathe Entonox in through a face mask which you hold yourself, thereby remaining in control of the amount you take. It is often found sufficient in itself.

Pethidine

This has an unpredictable effect. It may send you into a deep sleep, so that you miss the rest of your labour, or it may make you very confused. It may make your baby sleepy for a few days after the birth. This can disturb the relationship between you and make breastfeeding difficult. However, this might be preferable to being distressed because you cannot relax. The decision is yours.

What is happening   Pethidine is given by injection.

Helping yourself   Always ask for an internal examination before accepting pethidine. The labour may be almost over already. When you are sure in your own mind that you would benefit from it, ask for a small dose (for example 25 or 50 mg). It is a 'mood intensifier', so try to accept it cheerfully. Realize that you may need to make extra efforts to get the baby feeding properly afterwards.

Relaxation/breathing   Continue to use relaxation and breathing to help you.

Partner's help   Remind staff of your partner's wish to have an internal examination before accepting pethidine. If she is almost fully dilated, remind her that it is now too late for pethidine and support her through this climax of strong contractions.

Epidural

For most people this provides complete absence of sensation in the pelvic region. It can be useful in some specific situations, but if still effective in the second stage, pushing can be difficult and the baby may present awkwardly. This makes a forceps delivery more likely.

What is happening   A local anaesthetic is inserted into the epidural cavity of the spine by an anaesthetist. It may take as long as twenty or thirty minutes to take effect and you may need to be rolled on to one side or the other to spread the anaesthetic evenly. A drip into a vein in your arm will be set up, as a safeguard against your blood pressure dropping too low.

Helping yourself   Be certain that your situation calls for an epidural. Ascertain which stage of labour you have reached, or you may start pushing before the epidural takes effect. Ask for the epidural to wear off at the end of the first stage so that you can then push effectively.

Relaxation/breathing/position   Relax while the epidural is being performed, and breathe as necessary. Lie curled up on your side, or sit forward. Once the catheter is in place you can sit upright. When the midwife tells you there is a contraction, push as you have been shown in classes.

Partner's help   Ensure that it is not too late in the labour for this to be appropriate. Help her to relax and keep still when the anaesthetic is being administered. Help her to push effectively in the second stage.

If you have needed assistance with your labour and delivery, try to remember that this can affect your initial responses to your baby and his ability to respond to you. Allow time for recovery and for the perhaps more gradual development of feelings of attachment than you might have anticipated.

Complications

Any section on complicated labours is going to sound rather pessimistic and grim. As you read this, remember that statistically the chances are that your labour will be quite straightforward. However, since one never knows in advance what kind of labour is in store, it is best to learn about the common complications so that if you do happen to experience one or more of them you will be prepared and better able to cope.

Induction of labour

There are good reasons why labour sometimes needs to be induced, such as raised blood pressure, pre-eclampsia, diabetes, Rhesus incompatibility, and bleeding in late pregnancy. The reasons for induction should be explained to you and your willing consent to the operation should be obtained.

Many obstetricians do not like women to go past the expected date of delivery by more than a few days, and/or they like to induce labour if the diastolic blood pressure (the second figure of the recorded level, e.g. 130/95) exceeds 90 mm of mercury. However, other obstetricians doubt whether, if the mother is otherwise healthy, these are by themselves sufficient justifications to induce labour. If you are not satisfied with the reason given to you, you should insist on a further explanation.

If labour is to be induced, you may be asked to stay in hospital the night before the induction is planned. This is not essential: you could stay at home and arrive at the hospital early in the morning if you prefer. If your cervix is 'ripe' (soft, short, beginning to open, and the baby's head is in the pelvic cavity) labour may be induced by rupturing the membranes. You will be asked to empty your bladder and then to lie on a delivery bed with your hips and knees bent, your feet supported in stirrups and your legs apart. This is the lithotomy position. The doctor washes your vulva down with an antiseptic solution, confirms the state of the cervix and the position of the baby by a vaginal examination, and then makes a hole in the membranes bulging through the cervix (forewaters) with a pair of forceps passed along his fingers.

If the cervix is not ripe, induction is usually brought about by putting a needle into a vein in your arm so that a solution containing the hormone oxytocin can be dripped into your circulation at a controlled rate to make your uterus contract and open the cervix. Later on the membranes can be ruptured.

Some obstetricians always combine rupture of the membranes with the use of intravenous oxytocin to induce labour.

Prostaglandin pessaries or creams are sometimes used in the vagina to ripen the cervix as a preparation for induction, or as a means of inducing labour.

Bleeding in labour

Labour usually starts with a show of blood, which is the thick, sticky mucus plug from the cervix with some fresh or older blood. Continued fresh bleeding, however, is not normal. The reason for this may be that the placenta is placed abnormally low in the uterus (placenta praevia) and below the leading part of the baby. Under these circumstances the baby can only be born safely by delivery from above the placenta using Caesarean section.

If abnormal bleeding occurs when labour has begun and the position of the placenta is not already known from an ultrasound scan examination, a vaginal examination is made in an operating theatre, with preparations complete for Caesarean section, to feel whether or not the placenta is in the way. Depending on the degree of likelihood of placenta praevia being present, and therefore the need for a Caesarean section, you may be given a general anaesthetic for this examination.

Fetal distress

Fetal distress means that the baby is suffering from lack of oxygen. Warning that this may be happening is given by the passage of meconium from the baby's bowels so that the amniotic fluid (the liquid around the baby) is stained green or yellow, and by changes in the fetal heart-rate outside the normal limits of 120 to 160 beats per minute. If these warning signs occur, a fetal heart-rate monitor can be used to make a continuous recording of how the baby is reacting to the stress of labour.

If evidence of fetal distress persists or gets worse, action is usually taken to deliver the baby as soon as possible. If fetal distress occurs in the first stage of labour, before the cervix is fully dilated, Caesarean section is necessary. If it happens in the second stage of labour, depending on the position of the baby's head, delivery may be hastened by an episiotomy or by using forceps.

Some obstetricians will give you oxygen to breathe if signs of fetal distress appear or will ask you to lie on your side, since this increases the blood flow to the uterus. In some hospitals a sample of the baby's blood is obtained for gas analysis to find out whether the signs of fetal distress are caused by lack of oxygen or by another reason. This fetal blood sample is taken with you in the lithotomy position. A metal tube (amnioscope) is passed along the vagina and through the cervix to prick the baby's head. The drip of blood that oozes out is sucked up in a tube so that it can be analysed.

Prolapse of the umbilical cord   Fetal distress may also occur, and usually very suddenly, if the umbilical cord slips down and is compressed between the presenting part of the baby and your pelvic bones. The time when this is most likely to happen is when the waters break before the baby's head is engaged in the pelvis. If the cervix is not fully dilated, the baby can be delivered by Caesarean section. In the second stage of labour, the birth can be hurried along by making an episiotomy or by using forceps.

Cord entanglement   It is quite common for the umbilical cord to be looped loosely around the baby's body or neck. More rarely the cord is shortened so much by the entanglement that during contractions, particularly in the second stage, it may be pulled tight so that blood is unable to flow freely to the baby, causing distress. After the baby's head is born, if the cord is looped around the neck of the baby, it is usually quite easy to slip the baby through the loops. Otherwise, a tight cord can be cut between clamps, to stop it bleeding and free the baby.

Cephalo-pelvic disproportion

Disproportion means that the baby's head is too big to pass easily through the mother's bony pelvis, either because the baby is too big, the head being relatively larger than it should be, or because her pelvis is too small. This possibility may have been suspected before labour from your small stature, examination of the pelvis, or because the baby's head does not engage in your pelvis. The size of the baby's head can be measured using ultrasound, and the size of your pelvis can be measured on an X-ray. With disproportion, progress is slow and labour may stop. The only safe way to deal with this problem is by Caesarean section. If disproportion is suspected but not absolutely certain before your labour begins, a trial of labour may be conducted to see whether the baby can negotiate the birth canal reasonably, but everything will be ready to do a Caesarean operation should it prove necessary.

Abnormal positions of the head

In normal birth the top of the baby's head (the vertex) is the first part to appear. The baby has his chin tucked well into his chest so that he looks backwards to your spine and the back of his head lies towards your abdomen (occipito-anterior position). Sometimes, however, the baby's head is not in this usual position and steps must be taken to assist the birth.

Occipito-posterior position   When labour begins the back of the baby's head (occiput) usually points to one or other side, and only turns to the front as labour progresses and the head gets lower in the pelvis. Sometimes the back of the baby's head rotates towards your spine instead of forwards: this is an occipito-posterior position, and often means that labour is prolonged and that contractions tend to be less regular and to be associated with a lot of backache. In most women who start labour with an occipito-posterior position, rotation forwards does occur and the baby is delivered normally. If the woman kneels, supported on her knees and forearms, this often encourages the baby's head to rotate more quickly into the correct position.

If the occipito-posterior position persists, the baby can still be delivered normally with his face looking towards your abdomen: called a 'face-to pubes' delivery. On some occasions the baby's head fails to rotate completely and progress in the second stage is slowed right down because the baby's head can turn neither backwards nor forwards—it is stuck looking sideways (deep transverse arrest). This situation requires correction and delivery under anaesthesia by turning the baby's head with a hand, with forceps, or with the vacuum extractor (Ventouse).

Problems of head flexion If the baby's head is not well tucked into his chest (i.e. not fully flexed on the spine), the baby's head is not as small as it can be to pass down the birth canal. 'Moulding' normally occurs—that is, if the baby's head is presenting crown first, the head becomes long and narrow. However, if any other part of the head comes first, this may result in delay in labour, especially in the second stage. If deflexion occurs in the second stage—usually with an occipito-posterior position or deep transverse arrest—it is corrected at the same time as the fault in rotation, under anaesthesia. If the baby's head becomes still more deflexed so that the forehead is leading to give a *brow presentation*, labour is completely obstructed and delivery by Caesarean section is necessary. This is a very rare complication. More commonly, but still rarely, the baby's head is completely unbent on the spine so that the face actually leads and looks down the birth canal. *Face presentations* can be delivered normally although assistance may be necessary. Because the face takes all the pressure of labour, at birth it is swollen and bruised. This passes off within three to four days and leaves the baby without permanent damage and looking normal.

Breech presentation

Ninety-eight per cent of babies in the last few weeks before delivery settle to lie head downwards and are born this way. In the remainder the bottom or breech of the baby is the presenting part. Breech deliveries cause concern because the risks of delivery for the baby are greater than if the head comes first. This is because the head is the largest part of the baby and it has the most difficulty in passing through the pelvis. In normal labour the head has a long time to adapt and mould itself, whereas in breech delivery the head has to pass through the birth canal in a matter of a few minutes. This means that there is more chance of damage inside the baby's head if it passes through too quickly, whilst if there is delay in the birth of the head there is a greater chance that the baby will suffer from lack of oxygen.

For a breech delivery to be safe, therefore, the pelvis must be roomy. To be certain of this, X-ray pelvimetry (pelvic measurement) may be helpful, to find out whether vaginal delivery or Caesarean section would be the safer method of birth.

Because of the risks of breech delivery, some doctors try to turn babies so that they are head down before labour starts—*external cephalic version*. Others think that you succeed in turning only those who would have turned by themselves anyway. During the last eight weeks of pregnancy the baby may be encouraged to turn by the mother resting for about twenty minutes twice a day in a kneeling position, leaning down on her forearms on the floor (knee–chest position).

The first stage of labour is the same whether the head or breech presents. In the second stage, help and anaesthesia are more often required.

Twins

With two or more babies labour usually starts a week or two before the expected date of delivery. The first stage is as usual. The babies may be born head or breech first in almost any combination. There is usually a pause of 10–20 minutes between the birth of one baby and the next. The placenta is delivered after both babies are born.

Transverse lie

Rarely labour may start with the baby lying across your abdomen instead of either head or breech first. He cannot be delivered like this and so Caesarean section is usually required, unless before the membranes rupture he can be turned easily and nothing (like the placenta) is obstructing the passage through the cervix.

Unstable lie

Some babies even near the expected date of delivery may constantly change their position from head to breech presentations, to transverse lie. This sort of unstable lie is dangerous because it may be the result of obstruction to the birth canal, which requires special treatment. An unstable lie is also more likely to be associated with prolapse of the umbilical cord when the membranes rupture. For these reasons women with an unstable lie are often observed in hospital until the baby is born so that any unexpected complications can be dealt with immediately.

Forceps delivery

When the baby is presenting by the head, forceps are used to hasten delivery if there is fetal distress, if you become too tired or distressed, or if progress is too slow. Most obstetricians would regard two hours as the upper limit for a normal second stage in a first labour, and one hour if you are having your second or subsequent baby. Some obstetricians are more active than this and may regard half that time as long enough; however, recently published work has shown that, as long as the baby is not distressed, even as long as three or four hours does not do any harm.

Anaesthesia is required for forceps delivery: either general anaesthesia, epidural anaesthesia, or a pudendal block. A pudendal block is local anaesthetic injected around the vulva and into the vagina to numb the nerves supplying these parts. An episiotomy is usually done to make forceps delivery easier so that it causes less damage to your tissues and less force is applied to the baby.

Manual removal of the placenta

The placenta is usually delivered within 30 minutes of your baby's birth. If there is delay beyond this, or if at any time heavy bleeding occurs, the placenta can be removed by the doctor. A general anaesthetic is given (if you do not already have an epidural) and the doctor passes a hand along the vagina and into the uterus to separate the placenta with his fingers and then remove it.

How to cope with a Caesarean section

Some women need a surgical operation called a 'Caesarean section' to deliver their babies. If your doctor suggests during your antenatal care that a Caesarean section may be advisable, discuss this fully. Many couples want to be fully informed, to share in the decision-making and, if necessary, to ask for a second obstetric opinion. Sometimes, however, a Caesarean must be done for an unexpected reason, so it is worth knowing about Caesareans, even if you probably won't have one.

Traditionally the factors given consideration in labour are: the passenger (baby), the powers (uterine contractions), and the passages (the pelvis and its surrounding structures). A Caesarean birth is necessary when it is unsafe or difficult for the baby to be born vaginally. The reasons (see below) are not absolute, as is reflected by the very variable Caesarean section birth-rates. In this country the rate varies from region to region and hospital to hospital, the national average being 12.5 per cent. One French hospital quotes a rate of 5 per cent and in some parts of the USA the rate is as high as 30 per cent.

Reasons for a Caesarean birth

The passenger (the baby)   (a) Fetal distress, i.e. oxygen lack. This may be acute, for example due to partial or complete compression of the cord. (b) Placental insufficiency, which is a more prolonged form of oxygen lack which may become acute during labour.

The powers (uterine contractions)   Contractions may be present, but for some reason they are inefficient and perhaps irregular and the cervix (neck of the womb) dilates only a little or not at all (cervical dystocia). This may occur either in spontaneous labour or after induction.

The passages (the pelvis and its surrounding structures) These are termed mechanical difficulties, for example: (a) There may be a discrepancy between the size of the baby's head and the mother's pelvis (cephalo-pelvic disproportion); this is difficult to diagnose in a first pregnancy (except in extreme cases) until labour is underway. (b) There may be a large baby lying in the breech position. The size of the baby's head in relation to the size of the pelvis is particularly important in this instance, and whether to perform a Caesarean for breech births is often controversial. (c) The afterbirth may be low-lying (placenta praevia); there are degrees of this, and a Caesarean is only necessary when the placenta is lying right over the neck of the womb.

The mother A planned or elective Caesarean may also be performed if the mother has a condition such as diabetes, very high blood pressure, or detachment of the retina.

The need for a Caesarean may not be recognized until labour is underway, for example in the case of unexpected cephalo-pelvic disproportion or fetal distress. It is then that an emergency Caesarean birth is performed. If there is a previously diagnosed reason for a Caesarean birth it is described as planned or elective. This is usually performed a week or less before the expected date of delivery, or soon after the onset of spontaneous labour. Some mothers find the preparations for this, for example enema, shaving, and sometimes the removal of contact lenses, rather unpleasant when experienced 'cold'.

If there is any doubt about the need for a Caesarean, then you will have a trial of labour. This is particularly important if cephalo-pelvic disproportion is suspected, because it is only when labour is underway that the pelvis is properly 'tried'. If the contractions are efficient, then all the factors may work together to allow the baby's head to take up the optimum position for delivery. Also the pelvis itself is not a rigid structure, especially in late pregnancy, due to the effects of hormones. Depending on its shape, a small pelvis may well allow the head to pass through. The size of the outlet of the pelvis is also affected by the posture adopted. Trial of labour and careful monitoring are also important if there is placental insufficiency or if you have had a previous Caesarean birth. In this last instance the scar is also 'on trial'.

Which type of anaesthetic?

Epidural anaesthesia is increasingly available for Caesarean birth. It can only be given by anaesthetists, or by obstetricians with special experience, and therefore may not be available twenty-four hours a day in all hospitals. Sometimes epidural anaesthesia is not advisable for medical reasons, for example low blood pressure, any infection at the site of insertion, or back trouble. None of the anaesthetic dulls the brain and the mother remains awake and aware of the baby's birth. Many women have found that recovery, both physical and emotional, is quicker after an epidural than after a general anaesthetic. Also, the baby benefits from having less anaesthetic.

Some people prefer to be 'asleep' for the operation and this is a perfectly natural feeling. You should not be pressurized into having an epidural if you really do not want one. While all anaesthesia carries some risk, modern techniques have reduced this considerably and both types of anaesthetic are relatively safe for mother and baby. There may not be time to set up an epidural if the need for a Caesarean arises suddenly, as it takes about twenty to forty minutes. But a general anaesthetic can be given within minutes.

Preparing yourself

It is worth while going to antenatal classes, even if your Caesarean is planned in advance. You will learn how your body adapts during pregnancy, and practise relaxation and breathing techniques which will be useful before, during, and after the baby's birth. You will also be part of a group, sharing each other's anxieties, joys, and hopes, and you may be able to make friendships which will bring mutual support long after the birth. Your partner would also benefit from such participation.

Whichever type of anaesthetic you hope to have, stopping smoking will not only benefit your baby, but will also aid your recovery. If you think you may have a general anaesthetic, the following exercise will be useful afterwards and can be practised before the birth.

Place your hands on the sides of your lower ribs, breathe out with a little hiss for as long as you can, feeling your hands come together as you do it. Then breathe in, letting your ribs expand sideways. Repeat four times. Then take a deep breath in, let the breath out quickly, and cough as deeply as possible.

When you learn that a Caesarean section has been recommended for you, it is worth discussing several important points with the obstetrician, for example:

(a) Is a Caesarean birth really necessary?

(b) Which type of anaesthetic you would prefer. To help you make such a choice (if it exists) your GP, or local NCT teacher, can put you in touch with mothers who have experienced both.

(c) You may wish to point out that you would prefer a horizontal scar if this is possible.

(d) The role of your partner, as he can sometimes feel excluded at a Caesarean birth. He can usually be present during an epidural Caesarean and some hospitals allow him to be present if a general anaesthetic is given.

(e) Whether the baby will be left with you for as long as you want, providing he is healthy.

This may be a good time to request permission to take photographs of the birth, or to ask if someone else can do so. If the mother is having a general anaesthetic a photograph and/or the father's account of the birth can be an aid to bonding. If your partner has to wait outside the theatre, he can ask that the baby be brought to him after being checked by the paediatrician.

It is also important, if possible, to plan ahead for when you come out of hospital, remembering that you will not only have experienced the birth of a baby, but also had an abdominal operation. It is probably wise to aim for two weeks of extra help in the home from whatever source you can muster!

General anaesthetic

If the operation is planned you will go into hospital the day before and you will not be allowed to eat for at least six hours prior to the operation. You may be given an injection which will make your mouth feel dry. This is called a 'pre-med' but is given less often nowadays. Most mothers are given an antacid to drink which neutralizes stomach acidity, and you may have a tube passed through your nose to your stomach to ensure complete emptying of its contents.

Once in the theatre you may be given oxygen through a mask, which will help the baby. A catheter is passed to keep your bladder empty, and this may be done before or after you are anaesthetized. The anaesthetic is given initially by intravenous injection into your arm, and you will drift off to sleep within a minute or two. At some stage a drip will be set up and is likely to be still attached to your arm when you wake up. The catheter into your bladder may also still be in place at this stage.

Your baby will usually be born within the first ten minutes and the total operation may take twenty to forty minutes. The placenta (afterbirth) is delivered through the wound, and then the wall of the uterus and the other layers are carefully stitched. It is often a long wait for the father, so if all is well with the baby he can have first cuddle, and will be able to introduce you when you come round.

When you first wake up you may have considerable pain in your abdomen, and will not want to move at all. Before having a pain-killing injection try to cuddle your baby and offer the breast. Your partner can help with this as can the midwives. You may need injections for pain relief for the first twenty-four hours or so—only a small amount of the drug passes into the breast milk, and this has not been shown to harm the baby. It is important you have relief from pain if you need it, so that you can move about more easily and begin to handle and get to know your baby. Later, you can be given pain-relieving tablets, but do ask if you need them as they are not always offered. Conversely if you do not want them you can refuse.

Epidural anaesthetic

You will be asked either to sit upright with your feet over the edge of the bed, or to lie on your side. A small amount of local anaesthetic is injected into the skin of your lower back and then, when the area is numbed, a needle is inserted between two vertebrae into the epidural space (the area outside the coverings of the spinal cord). You may feel a sharp pain as the needle goes in—remember your relaxation techniques. A fine plastic tube is then threaded through the needle and stays in place when the needle is withdrawn. A syringe is attached to the other end of the tube and the local anaesthetic injected. After a while your lower abdomen and legs will become numb. You may be asked to turn from side to side to spread the anaesthetic. Your legs may become weak and some women cannot move them at all. A drip will be set up and your blood pressure frequently checked.

In the operating-theatre your lower body will be screened from your view. Your partner will sit at your side and neither of you will see the operation site. Although you will not feel pain you may feel a peculiar stretching sensation during the operation. Both of you will see your baby as soon as he is born and hear the first cry. Once the paediatrician has checked the baby briefly you or your partner may be able to hold the baby until the operation is completed.

The three of you should be able to spend some time together undisturbed once the operation is over and you can offer the baby your breast. You will be pain-free until the epidural wears off and you may be able to have a further top-up dose to see you through the first hours. Ask about this possibility, or say if you would prefer not to.

As the epidural wears off, the movement and sensation will gradually return to your legs and abdomen, and you can have a

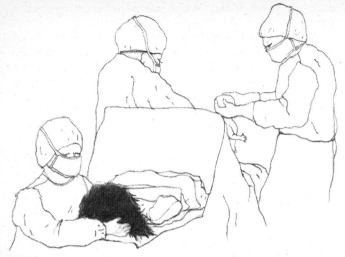

Typical screening for epidural Caesarean birth

pain-killing injection if you wish. Some mothers need one only at night.

In the ward

Initially you will have a drip in your arm, which will be removed once you have started drinking (usually in 12–24 hours). Passing urine may be painful the first time—relaxation and steady breathing can help. Although it seems cruel, you will soon be asked to get out of bed, as mobility improves your circulation and aids your general recovery. Whilst you are in bed, remember to wriggle your toes and move your feet as much as possible. A physiotherapist will help you with breathing, and show you how to support your scar in order to cough. You will need to support it in order to sneeze and laugh as well!

Your wound will be covered with a small dressing. A few people also have a fine plastic tube which drains any excess fluid from the wound. This is usually removed after one or two days. The wound is inspected daily, and the dressing remains on as long as necessary. Occasionally a self-dissolving stitch is used.

Like all women who have given birth, you will have a vaginal discharge; this is usually red at first, and then gradually changes to brown and then pink. This is called 'lochia' and will continue for anything between one and four weeks. Anything which rubs over the area of the scar is uncomfortable, so it is usually best to use waist-high stretch pants to hold the towels in place rather than sanitary belts. Slip-on slippers or sandals are a must, as you cannot reach your feet!

You will have a lot of rumbling in your tummy for a few days and may pass a lot of wind. Peppermint water can ease this. Don't be discouraged or alarmed if you have considerable pain over the site of your wound. Remember that pain-killers are available and that each day sees you further on the road to recovery. For the first three to four days you will be given a light diet, but you will soon be able to eat normally. Often a suppository or an enema is offered routinely on the second or third day to help with passing wind, but you do not need to accept it if all is well. If after a few days you have difficulties having your bowels open, ask for a laxative.

Breastfeeding

It is perfectly possible to breastfeed after a Caesarean. Sometimes it is more difficult to establish than after a vaginal birth, especially if mother or baby is sleepy after a general anaesthetic. Even so, with early frequent suckling your milk will 'come in'. As your tummy will be sore, you will need extra help getting the baby into a good position. Do not hesitate to ask staff or other mothers to lift your baby out of the crib for you whenever he cries.

If you have a vertical scar (a) Sit up and put a pillow on one side of you. Rest the baby's head on it with his feet over your thighs. There is then less strain involved in holding the baby up. (b) Lay the baby on a pillow with his head facing the breast and feed him lying under your arm. This leaves both arms free to lift the

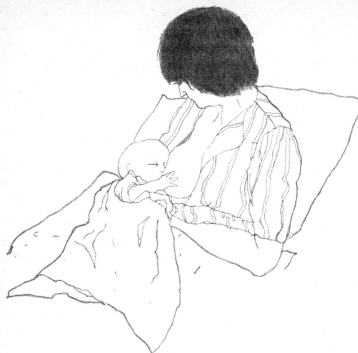

Breastfeeding—vertical scar

baby's head to the breast. Sit straight to avoid straining your tummy. (c) Lay your baby on a pillow on top of the meal table which fits over the bed.

If you have a horizontal scar (a) Sit up and lay pillows horizontally across your stomach and feed normally. (b) Use the meal table as described in (c) above. (c) Lie down on the bed on your side with the baby beside you and feed him facing you.

Do ask the ward sister for help if you have any difficulties. If this is not forthcoming in hospital, ask a friend or relative to contact the local NCT breastfeeding counsellor. She can also visit you at home if you need her.

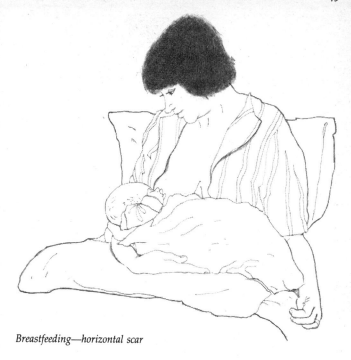

Breastfeeding—horizontal scar

Occasionally babies have to go to the special care unit. If you are distressed by this, be sure and ask if it is absolutely necessary. Make sure the staff know that you want to breast-feed. If your baby is unable to suckle at the breast at first, ask for help to express your milk. This can then be fed to your baby who gets the benefit of your milk and it also ensures that your supply gets established.

Try to visit the unit as soon and as much as possible—the baby needs to hear your voice and feel your touch from the first day, if possible. If the unit is a long way from your ward ask for a wheelchair so that your partner or a nurse can take you down. Having a photograph of the baby by your bed can help to lessen the feeling of separation.

Getting out of bed

Your first challenge will be getting out of bed. Some hospital beds can be lowered, which is a great help. If yours cannot, ask for a footstool.

(a) Push your palms into the bed close to your sides and lift your bottom. Repeat this until you reach the left side of the bed. Then imagine yourself to be a string puppet. With both hands lift your left knee and place your left foot on the footstool (or floor), then lift the right knee so that you can ease yourself out of bed. Do *not* try to lift a *whole* leg from the hip. (b) You can shift your legs to the side of the bed by waggling one foot sideways (heel–toes) and then doing the same with the other until your legs are together; then sit upright on the edge of the bed.

However you do it: *Take your time, breathe long, gentle, slow breaths, and do everything yourself.*

You may be asked on the first day to get out of bed while it is made, so remember the above 'rules' and avoid the assistance of someone who may try to pull you forward only to let you drop back again, which would be very painful for you.

Getting into bed

Vertical section Face the side of the bed, climb on to the footstool and then on to the bed on all fours, turn and 'reverse' well up back against the pillows. To inch your way from perching sideways on the bed is slower and more uncomfortable.

Horizontal section Sit well back on to the bed with your back against the pillows and then slowly lift and slide your legs on to the bed, and lift your bottom into the pillows by pushing down with your palms.

After the first few days, if you slip down in bed and need propping up, you can hold on to the bar, or bedhead, above you and this will take all the strain while you tuck your bottom against the pillows. Dig your heels into the sheets.

Walking

Stand up as straight as possible so that gravity does not pull the weight of your abdominal contents against the scar. Support your tummy and use the breathing taught for labour and move from bed to chair as though this were a contraction. Calm breathing is helpful to relax you before breastfeeding and after walking or moving about; it prevents you remaining tense because of abdominal pain.

Sitting

Choose hard upright chairs, if possible with arms. Put one leg behind the other, *bend your knees* to take the strain—then sit. Do this to get up too, rather than planting two feet together. If your chair has no arms, sit on one buttock and edge back sideways.

Using the lavatory

You may be asked to use the lavatory on the first day. Again, use bent knees to take the strain and hold on to any rails nearby. Relax your pelvic floor and the muscles of your face (which are associated with the pelvic floor muscles) to help the flow of urine. A bidet may be available for washing the area of your genitals: remember to check temperatures—you won't be able to leap up if the bidet feels cold or the water feels too hot! Use the bidet to wash your feet as well if you want to.

Getting to know your baby

Probably you will feel strongly about your baby right from the start, but some of you may find it hard to realize that the baby in the cot beside you is actually 'yours'—especially if you had a general anaesthetic and were therefore not aware of the birth. Spend as much time holding and talking to your baby as you can. Breastfeeding is a real help in this situation. Sometimes family likeness (especially in old baby photographs) helps to convince you that this is really your baby.

Many women, regardless of the way they give birth, do not have strong maternal feelings straight away—it takes time to get to know your baby whatever sort of delivery you have had. If there are other mothers in your ward who have had Caesareans, ask if you can be together. You will probably find they feel the same as you do, and discussing your feelings and worries can help a great deal. Don't be upset by mothers who have had vaginal births who think you have 'opted for the easy way out'.

At home

You will probably stay in hospital for between six and ten days. Although you may feel quite fit in this environment do not be surprised if you feel a bit 'wobbly' when you get home. Remember you have had a major operation as well as the emotional experience of giving birth! It is sometimes particularly hard for you if you had a long labour before your Caesarean birth. Take things as easily as you can—take one day at a time and gradually over the first month you will feel stronger.

Concentrate on caring for the baby and yourself and cut the housework to the bare essentials. Most of it will wait. If help is offered, accept it. Be especially careful about lifting heavy objects. If you must lift, remember to bend your knees, keep your back straight, and face directly the object to be lifted. Increase your postnatal exercises gradually.

Don't be surprised if it takes at least a month to recover. The local NCT teacher will probably be able to put you in touch with others who have had Caesarean births: it can be helpful to discuss your physical and emotional feelings with others who have had Caesareans. Postnatal depression can occur after any type of birth. If you feel low or are having problems relating to your baby, do discuss this with your partner and do ask for help from your family doctor, midwife, health visitor, NCT post-natal group, or Caesarean Support Group.

Getting back to normal

Your scar will gradually feel less sore and may then become itchy. It sometimes remains sensitive for a while and in appearance will gradually fade from red to brown to white. Pants that come up to your waist are more comfortable initially and loose clothes are essential.

Lovemaking can be resumed as soon as you feel ready, though you may need to experiment with positions which do not put pressure on your scar. Do remember to use some form of contraception—methods can be discussed while you are in hospital and reviewed at your six-week check-up. You will not be able to have a coil fitted for three months.

Just as those who have had vaginal deliveries are sometimes concerned that lovemaking 'might not be the same as before', some women, especially those who have a vertical scar, are worried that their partner will find their changed appearance off-putting. Sharing your feelings and talking openly with your partner can help to sort out these anxieties.

What about the future?

Once you have had a Caesarean birth, all future labours should take place in hospital, as there is some risk of the uterine scar-tissue breaking down. It is quite possible to have a vaginal birth following a Caesarean, but this does tend to depend on why it was done in the first place. For instance, if you needed a Caesarean because of placenta praevia, fetal distress, or because the baby was in the breech position, then you would not normally need an operative delivery in your next pregnancy. However, if your baby was delivered by Caesarean because of a small or unfavourably shaped pelvis, then a Caesarean needs to be repeated for subsequent births. An X-ray of your pelvis may be arranged after a Caesarean birth to determine its size and shape as this can give some guide as to the outcome of future pregnancies. Thus it is important that before you leave hospital you speak to the doctors involved to ascertain why the Caesarean was necessary and whether it will be essential for future births.

Episiotomy

Episiotomy is the surgical enlargement of the birth outlet, used to prevent over-stretching of the pelvic floor and to enable the baby to be born easily and without tearing the muscles of the mother's pelvic floor. In some hospitals episiotomies are routine with first babies. However, a mother who can relax her pelvic floor and work with the midwife during the delivery of her baby is less likely to need an episiotomy than a mother who is tense, and the ability to adopt a semi-upright or upright position can also work in your favour.

Some doctors and midwives feel that far too many routine episiotomies are done nowadays. Until the last decade or so, midwives were taught to deliver babies so that episiotomies were rare and a mother's intact perineum was a tribute to the midwife's skill. Then episiotomies became medically fashionable to prevent damage to the mother's tissues, to avoid later prolapse of the uterus (although neither of these claims has been substantiated), and to give a 'nice tight vagina' for subsequent sexual intercourse. A recent survey on episiotomy (Sheila Kitzinger for the NCT) showed that many women found the scar from an episiotomy interfered with their sex life for many months, sometimes years. The pendulum is swinging again and there are doctors who now believe that a second-degree tear (one involving skin, and the underlying muscle fibre) is often preferable to an episiotomy, because the tear is limited by need and not by the judgement of the midwife or obstetrician who is making the cut with a pair of scissors. They feel that prolapses are less common now that women are better fed and have fewer children, and that some episiotomies are performed with inadequate anaesthesia and repaired badly.

There are, obviously, cases where episiotomy is very necessary for the sake of both mother and baby. But it is a good idea, at your antenatal visits, to discuss your hospital's policy about episiotomy and make your own views known to those who will be taking care of you. Tell them again when you are in labour.

What to do before the baby is born

Suitable exercises which increase the voluntary control of the muscles and increase the blood supply to the pelvic floor to improve its condition and healing property are:

Tighten and relax the muscles controlling the passage of urine (practise this while urinating—three or four times on each occasion).

Tighten and relax the ring of muscles around the anus.

Raise and lower the pelvic floor, imagining it to be a lift in a building, slowly going up, going down again, down into the basement (bulging out the vagina) and drawing up to the ground floor again.

Make smooth movements with the vaginal muscles, as though rolling them around a tennis ball (clockwise and then counter-clockwise); or imagine writing or drawing with a pencil held in the vagina.

(Note: the latter sets of exercises need not involve any movement of the thigh muscles—the legs should be slightly apart and the exercises may be practised while sitting, lying, standing, or kneeling.)

Practise a delivery position, half-lying with your upper back and head supported on several pillows, knees bent with the feet resting on the bed, hip-width apart and with the knees allowed to flop outwards. Sit with the weight on the base of your spine, not on your buttocks.

Practising for the delivery of the baby's head and shoulders should be done with relaxed thigh muscles and mouth, to help relax the vagina. Smiling helps many people to relax.

The episiotomy

A local anaesthetic will be given in advance if it is obvious that an episiotomy (see also p. 125) will be needed, since it takes several minutes before the tissues are numbed. If it is done during delivery to prevent tearing, the cut is made at the peak of a contraction when the nerve endings are numbed by the stretching. In either case, the mother should be aware only of stretching caused by the pressure of the baby's head and then sudden relief as the episiotomy enlarges the opening and the baby's head slips out. If it is done as an emergency procedure it may not be possible to ensure the mother's comfort, but she can reassure herself that although it hurt, it was done quickly and to help her and her baby. It should not be done until the baby's head is well down on the mother's perineum.

After an episiotomy, stitching will be necessary. More local anaesthetic should be given especially if there is a delay in suturing. If the stitching is painful, you should tell the doctor and say that the anaesthetic has not yet taken effect. If only one or two stitches are necessary you may be offered gas and oxygen rather than an injection. Nowadays the midwife may do the stitching.

Coping with the stitches

Some kinds of stitches dissolve after five or six days, others need to be removed when the cut has healed, again usually after five or six days. Some mothers experience few problems with stitches. However, for those who are uncomfortable or bruised, the following suggestions may be helpful.

Lie on your tummy, or half-lie on your back or side; it may be easier than sitting. For relief of discomfort, some hospitals recommend warm salt baths; some suggest using a bidet; still others suggest swabbing the pelvic area. As water can break down the scar, never spend very long in the bath; short, more frequent baths are better.

Sit well back on the lavatory: this helps to prevent urine stinging sore tissues. Hold the stitched area firmly with a clean pad when opening your bowels. Use soft toilet paper rather than hard (take your own to hospital if necessary).

Wear a sanitary belt to hold your pads, since this will provide firmer support than the sanitary pants into which pads can be inserted. Fairly tight stretch pants can be very comfortable, but pants which allow movement of the pad as you walk will rub the stitches. Resist the temptation to use talcum powder because it is known to irritate the ovaries. Self-adhesive pads will also rub in this way. Once the stitches have been removed, it may also be far more comfortable to use two-layer, soft paper-filled sanitary pads rather than the harsher paper-cotton wool types.

Some mothers have found homoeopathic remedies helpful in reducing shock and bruising and speeding healing. Tablets may be taken by mouth, or a tincture applied directly to the affected area. See p. 286.

For breastfeeding, you may find side-lying the most comfortable position; if your underneath elbow is raised on a pillow, it is easier for the baby to feed from the nipple. Take care to see that your breast is not compressed against the chest-wall, as this may lead to engorgement. Other suggestions for comfortable breastfeeding are to sit in an upright chair or to sit upright in bed, but on one buttock instead of on your whole bottom (or with one leg bent and the foot tucked up underneath your bottom), with the baby on a pillow under your arm.

Healing

A carefully stitched episiotomy should heal neatly, though you may find it very tender and painful for the first week, and occasionally uncomfortable for some weeks or even months after that.

Pelvic floor exercises should be started as soon as possible after the birth, and repeated frequently each day. After the delivery you can practise stream-stopping when passing urine, and gentle up-and-down movements of the whole pelvic floor, at any time. As the soreness decreases you can isolate the muscle movements and increase them in strength. Emphasis should now be put on tightening the muscles around the vagina and holding them tight for a count of four before relaxing.

You may find it reassuring to look at the pelvic floor with a hand mirror before the birth to see that there is space for the incision, and afterwards to see how small an area has been stitched.

Making love again

The problems of making love after an episiotomy are discussed on p. 248, but to sum up:

There is no magical date after which it is 'all right' to make love. The ideal time is when both partners desire it, regardless of the baby's age. Your pelvic floor muscles may be sore or tight following stitches, but waiting will not make them stretch. Your husband may be just as afraid of hurting you as you are afraid of being hurt; plenty of love-play before intercourse, with each having consideration for the other, helps to dispel any fear. Lubrication with special creams or jellies will make penetration more comfortable.

Bonding—developing early relationships with the baby

Bonding is the word which has recently been used to describe the developing relationship between mothers—or fathers —and their newborn babies. This relationship is a two-way process: the baby getting to know his parents, and the parents the child. It has been compared to courtship, it goes on over a long period of time, and it is unique to each pair of people. Many of its aspects are unlike any other human relationship, but there are also features which are not so different from a relationship, say, between a man and a woman in love.

What do parents want to know about bonding? What do they need to know about it? Chiefly, perhaps, to trust their own feelings.

Nearly every woman finds that as soon as her baby is born, she wants to hold him and to see and touch, at last, the baby which has been a part of her for so many months. The classic sketch of parents counting their baby's fingers and toes has always been a source of amusement, but it reflects a real and natural impulse, and parents who have been unable to hold their babies soon after birth have often felt unhappy about it at the time and for long afterwards. Some mothers who have held one child soon after its birth but had another child taken away, for whatever reason, have felt that it was easier for them to feel a sense of 'belonging' with the child held early than with the child taken away.

Recent research has demonstrated that this long-held feeling about the value of early holding of the newborn baby by his mother is founded on a good basis of fact. Research has been done, for instance, which suggests that the first hour and a half after a baby is born is a time of particular sensitivity and alertness in mother and baby, and that if the baby and its mother are not together during any of this time, then it may take extra effort for the 'bonding' process to proceed. Interest in this field of research arose from animal research (some mammals actually reject their offspring if not given contact immediately, although this is not true of human beings) and has been followed by careful research with human beings. This showed in particular that mothers who held their babies for an hour as soon as they were born and for extra time (in comparison with the other mothers in the study) on each of the next few days, established close relationships with their babies sooner than mothers given less contact. Two years later the mothers who had experienced extended contact used more questions, more adjectives and fewer commands, and at five years old their children scored better on language tests.

This kind of research has led all those working in maternity and paediatric care, or interested in parent–child relationships, to acknowledge the importance of the bonding process and to give special help in the cases where the mother and baby must be separated. It should be stressed that bonding is not something that has to be *done to* mothers and babies, but that it is a part of the process by which the new life assimilates the world. It is part of the long journey from fertilized egg to independent individual and ought not to be disrupted. Hospital routines which put babies into nurseries for almost all the time and bring them to their mothers only for clock-controlled feedtimes are an example of patterns to avoid: fortunately this attitude towards the care of mothers and babies is now rare. Of course the mother should not become over-tired, but she should be able to be with her baby as much as she likes and to share the baby with her husband, too.

Pregnancy

When a woman becomes pregnant there are things about her that will affect how she will behave with her baby: such things as her genetic inheritance from her own parents, her upbringing and education, her relationship with the child's father, and her beliefs about child-rearing practices. These and other factors will influence—and be influenced by—her actual experiences during pregnancy, labour, delivery, and then living with the baby.

Love between two adult individuals can be a mixture of many emotions, just as it can be between parents and children. The love of a parent for a child encompasses many facets including tenderness, protectiveness, and a powerful sense of belonging. Not all these emotions may be aroused at once, and there seems to be a great variation in when mothers first feel love for their babies. Some feel it first in pregnancy itself (especially when they first feel the baby move), some at the baby's birth, and some during the first few weeks after delivery. (The father, too, may find that his love does not come instantly, but grows and develops as he and the baby get to know one another.) The feelings of mother-love in pregnancy may be mingled with other feelings, such as fear or anxiety about whether the baby will be perfect.

During pregnancy there are already strong influences between the mother and her baby: hormonal changes caused by the baby's presence alter the mother's physiology, emotions, and behaviour. Her behaviour and emotions will in turn affect the baby's behaviour, probably via further hormones crossing from her blood across the placenta to the baby. External things will also influence the baby's behaviour inside the uterus: the sound of the blood flow through her uterus, loud noises, alterations in her position, light getting across the thin wall of her abdomen and uterus—all these will be appreciated by the unborn child. Perhaps the baby towards the end of pregnancy has already grown familiar with some aspects of her, such as the individual rhythms and variations of her heartbeat, which he may remember after birth.

Birth and afterwards

A woman's experience of childbirth is also likely to affect how her relationship with her baby develops, although this is not a matter of simple cause and effect: even the most strenuous, unusual, or painful labour can be the beginning of a firm 'bonding' if the mother makes it as positive an experience as she can.

Immediately after birth, particularly if no pain-killing drugs have been given, the mother and baby appear to go through a period of especial alertness lasting up to an hour and a half. It would seem natural that as far as possible, mothers, fathers, and babies should be together in close contact during this time. The baby in the mother's arms has the advantage of being warm and being kept near the breast. If he suckles the breast, he will aid the let-down reflex and help with the third stage of labour. The baby will also be near the comforting sound of the mother's heartbeat, and by being in close contact with her will be beginning to learn new features about her: her face, her voice, her smell, and her behaviour. From the parents' point of view this early contact with their baby may help them in their developing relationships with the child, and may have positive influences on their behaviour later on. For this reason—that it may in some way facilitate their relationship—mothers should be helped to have early contact with their babies whenever possible. However, where a very small or sick baby has to be taken away to have further care, the immediate physical health of the baby is of prime importance. After all, most relationships of any kind suffer temporary setbacks but are picked up again and developed at a later stage, ideally with the help of those around and concerned.

For human beings there is obviously no right or wrong way to behave with a baby immediately after birth, and from observations done in delivery rooms and at home births, there is every kind of variation. However, there do appear to be some kinds of behaviour which occur more often than others. For instance, there is a tendency for the mother to touch the baby first with her finger-tips—very gently and tentatively—then to stroke the baby with her fingers, and then to touch and move the limbs. There also appears to be an interest in the baby's eyes, with verbal encouragement to open them, and then a direct greeting of the baby when he does. Some mothers have reported that they do not really feel that the baby is alive until he has opened his eyes. Many mothers in this period also compare some feature of the baby with the baby's father, if he is present.

What of the baby during these moments? He may not go through such a long period of alertness for several further days. If he is in his mother's arms he may gaze into her face, for the newborn baby is particularly responsive to the features of human beings and, held in this position, his face is about nine inches away from his mother's face—the distance at which he can see best. He is also responsive to the sound of the human voice, especially slightly higher frequencies, which may explain why people tend to raise the pitch of their voices when talking to babies.

The first few months

Over the first weeks and months, the parents and the baby continue to learn, understand, and respond to one another's needs. The mother has to develop a new pattern of responsibility, covering 24 hours a day of feeding, cuddling, changing, cleaning, and talking to her child—and an infinite number of other responses. The father likewise finds that his role changes. It has been shown that fathers who are present at their children's births and who help to look after their babies immediately after birth, continue to offer support and practical help with care: they too have become bonded.

The baby, meanwhile, is learning about his parents. By six days of age he is able to distinguish between the smell of his own mother and the smell of a stranger; by ten days he seems able to distinguish between the caring ways of his own mother and those of a stranger. From early days he will respond differently to the sight of his own mother's face and to the sound of her voice, than to the face and voice of a stranger. Thus even this early, the baby—having been born with the ability to be more attracted to human beings than to objects in the environment—has become even more specific and has learned to respond particularly to his own parents: in fact, he has become bonded to them.

If separation does occur

Sometimes separation of the mother and baby is unavoidable: special care of mother or baby may be required, for instance, if the birth has been long or complicated, if an assisted delivery or Caesarean section has been required, or if the baby is ill or premature. It is important in such cases to remember that these mothers and babies will nevertheless develop their own relationship, starting whenever they can, and that some initial separation is not an irreparable 'bad start'. The bonding process is best facilitated by enabling mother and baby to have as much time together as possible, as soon as possible, but in human beings it is fortunately not absolutely dependent on a particular time or pattern. If you and your baby must be separated, do not be discouraged but do make every opportunity to be together, to look at the baby, to help with his care whenever possible, and to begin the bonding process as soon as you can, giving extra attention then in cuddles, holding, talking, singing, rocking, relaxing, and feeding. If the separation is to be prolonged, you may like to take a hint from special care baby units which give each mother a photograph of her baby to keep with her while the baby is in special care. Should the mother's illness be the cause of the separation, then the father can be the one to spend extra time with his new baby.

Many new parents feel awkward with their babies at first —whether the first contact is immediately at the baby's birth or delayed somewhat—and need to allow themselves time to get to know each other. Just as some friendships start very quickly, like 'falling in love at first sight', and some others take longer to form, like a good wine maturing or a green fruit ripening, so some parents very quickly feel a powerful sense of connection with their babies, while others develop this feeling more slowly. Many factors are involved, and there is no magic formula which results in instant bonding, nor any hard-and-fast rules which must be followed, nor even any typical pattern: you and your baby will form, given time together, a special relationship which is yours alone.

THE NEW
BABY

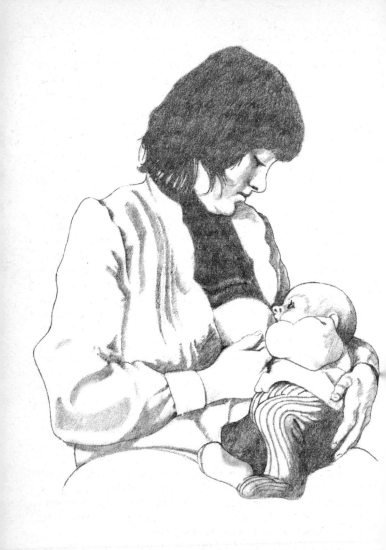

Introduction

Watching your baby grow and develop new skills is one of the most rewarding pleasures of parenthood, although of course it is wrong to be so obsessed with the next milestone that you ignore present achievements. We are recognizing how many skills even newborn babies possess, and they are no longer written off as helpless and passive little creatures.

Breastfeeding can be the most convenient and mutually satisfying way of feeding a baby. If you decide to breastfeed, it will be helpful for you to learn the theory beforehand. It would be reasonable to suppose that breastfeeding comes instinctively to the mother, but this does not necessarily happen. For thousands of years women watched one another feeding babies and learned, perhaps subconsciously, how it was done: what positions were most comfortable, what to do when there were physical snags, and so on. In one British community it was the custom for nursing mothers to wear a blue thread which had been handed down from mother to daughter through several generations. Ostensibly this was to ward off mastitis, but it must have acted as a tangible moral support: 'If my mother can do it, so can I.' However, nowadays the sight of a nursing mother is quite rare and women are thrown back on to their own resources to find out about the process of lactation.

If, for some reason, you cannot breastfeed your baby, or do not wish to do so, feel confident that the artificial milks available today are more satisfactory than their predecessors were. Whatever method of feeding you choose, the most important thing is to ensure that feedtimes are loving and happy occasions.

When your baby is about four to six months old he will probably like to start a mixed diet of milk and solids. It is quite unnecessary to spend a lot of money on commercially prepared baby food (other than for convenience) since the baby can easily eat modified versions of the family's meals.

This book does not set out to tell you exactly how to care for your baby, since the way you choose to do this will be individual to you, your personality and your circumstances. A few general hints, however, may apply to most people.

Some parents have specialized problems, if their babies are born prematurely or are handicapped in some way. Modern paediatric medicine can now do a great deal to help these children.

The parents of twins have to cope with the mixed blessings of a 'package-deal family' and may find it helpful to discover how best to cut corners and adapt their lives to the extra demands twin babies make.

Adoptive parents require information about infant feeding and basic babycare, too, and have special emotional needs as well, particularly during the period before the adoption is finalized.

The development of your baby from birth to one year old

'Is it all right?' is the first question asked by most new parents.

The midwife (or doctor, if there is one present) is concerned first to ascertain that your baby's head, spine, and limbs appear normal, and this is done at a glance. At the same time she will check to see that breathing begins within a minute or so and that the baby is a good colour, indicating that the heart and circulation are going well. She will also see that he is lively and that his muscle 'tone' is not too floppy. Sometimes the condition of the baby is rated by Apgar score (named after the doctor who devised it), in which each of five headings is checked and given a score of 0, 1, or 2; they are heart-rate, respiratory effort, muscle tone, colour, and reflex irritability. The assessment is made at one and five minutes after birth, the important thing being that there should be some improvement in the total score by the time of the second check.

During the first 24 hours your baby will have a full examination by the doctor, who will check every detail. At this time less obvious problems are identified, such as an unstable ('clicking') hip, minor degrees of cleft palate, undescended testicle, etc. If any treatment is required, arrangements can be made for this at once.

The brand-new baby

The newborn baby has a strong sucking reflex and it is advantageous to put your baby to the breast as soon as practicable after the birth, while the sucking response is strong. The baby has a 'rooting' reflex which means that when touched on the cheek by the breast, he will turn his head instinctively towards the touch.

The newborn baby will grasp tightly an object placed in his palm or curl his toes when touched on the sole. The 'walking reflex' which makes him lift his feet alternately if held just standing on a table is very strong in the first days, gradually diminishing in the first few weeks.

He will respond sharply to a sudden noise, but will be soothed by a gentle rhythmic sound. The baby will respond to voices directly in front of him and especially to his mother's voice.

The baby can distinguish the outline of something in front of him. He can focus at about nine inches but will not hold the gaze for more than a few seconds.

The first month

Your baby may smile from the first few days but the responsive smile tends to appear from four weeks onwards.

Sleeping patterns differ widely; one baby will sleep much in the day, waking only to be fed and changed, while another will sleep very little, perhaps only a few hours. It is important to play with your baby, talk to him and cuddle him when he is awake. Babies carried close to their mothers, especially in chest-to-chest contact, often seem more contented than babies who are left alone.

At some times the baby may wave his arms and legs happily, but will do this more strongly when unwrapped and placed on a cold surface, often crying unhappily. You may notice this when he is placed on a cold plastic changing mat or in the cold scales at the baby clinic.

When laid on his tummy, he can turn his head from side to side, and when held against your shoulder he may hold his head clear of your shoulder for a moment. His hands are curled with the thumb inwards. During this month he will uncurl from the fetal position.

Two to three months

His hands are now open and he will start to discover his hands and feet. He will be delighted to discover the relation between grasping the beads across the pram and hearing the rattling noise they make. He will kick his legs in the air. He will be able to grasp an object when given it and will grab at your hair or beads or glasses.

When lying on his tummy he will raise his head and shoulders up from the mattress. He can now roll from his side on to his back.

He will look long and hard at things around him, especially his mother's face. He will respond more positively to speech, becoming quiet or kicking and gurgling happily. Now he really enjoys a time of play on the rug or a large bed. Talk to him and sing and give him the opportunity to 'talk back'.

Three to six months

Now he may be able to roll over from front to back. He will enjoy taking his weight on his feet and being bounced gently.

He will begin to sit up supported and will look around with great interest. When placed on his front, he will raise his whole chest from the floor or mattress and hold this position. He may now begin to draw his knees up under his body and rock.

He tries to work out how to grasp his feet and is delighted when he succeeds. He will reach out for objects and grasp them firmly. He needs to be allowed to work out how to reach objects and you should not place them in his hand. He only copes with one object at a time. He will accept strangers happily, especially if you are present.

Six months to a year

Your baby will now be able to sit up unsupported. He will probably be crawling, though some babies never crawl but shuffle along on their bottoms, sometimes with one leg tucked underneath; they usually start later than crawlers and also walk later, perhaps not until 18 months.

During this period he will start to pull himself on to his feet and then move around holding on to the furniture, stepping sideways. He will stand up with support or alone, and by one year many babies will take their first steps alone.

He now enjoys toys which make a noise (squeak or hoot, for instance), and will be happy banging a spoon on a saucepan or putting objects into containers. He has learned to release his grasp as the grasp reflex disappears, so he throws his toys away and will give objects to you.

He will watch animals and machines with interest. He recognizes members of the family and well-known friends approaching from 20 feet or more away. He will know his own name and turn when he hears it.

He can understand most of what is said relating to his daily life and he babbles loudly, tunefully and incessantly. He can repeat syllables in long strings.

He imitates adults' sounds and actions, such as 'pat-a-cake' and waving 'bye-bye', and enjoys playing 'peep-bo'.

He can drink from a cup and will try to feed himself with a spoon. He is now chewing his food.

He clearly distinguishes strangers from family, and may hide his face and cling to you when a stranger approaches.

The health visitor

When the baby is about a fortnight old, your health visitor will call. She is a nurse who has had special training in the care and development of babies and new mothers, and her first job is to answer your questions—any questions, about anything. To do with feeding perhaps, or when to pick the baby up, how much to play with him, why his motions have changed colour, where to get supplementary benefit, what the doctor meant about clicking hips, etc. She works closely with your GP and they will often collaborate on any problem you or your baby may have. The health visitor runs the clinic where you take the baby for medical check-ups and immunizations, and will keep in touch with you until your child is five years old. She may also run a weekly mother-and-baby group for first-time mothers.

Going to the clinic

In every area there are clinics to which you can take your baby for regular checks and immunizations. Because it is also a good opportunity to meet other mothers, your visit to the clinic may become a pleasant social event! Arrangements vary a little, but your health visitor will give you all the local details.

At the clinic, the baby will be weighed and you can see the progress in his growth. Of course, some babies are bigger than others, but there is a 'range of normal', and special charts have been designed which outline this range—separate ones for boys and girls, who differ in growth rate from a surprisingly early age. You will see that the chart also shows the normal rate of growth for a baby. This is a very important factor. After a few visits you will be able to check that your baby is growing at a normal rate.

Examinations will be carried out to check that the baby is developing and that he is able to do the things expected of a child of his age. Again, there is a range of normal and the tests will show if the baby is within this range. The ages at which tests for these developmental changes are done may differ from one area to the next, but are usually at about two months and eight months, when the hearing is also tested.

Your baby as an individual

All the talk about 'normal' should not make you think that your baby is just like all the others—he is unique. From the moment he is conceived he is an individual in his own right and you will have the joy of watching him develop a personality and physique which are entirely his own. The summaries above of what to expect will help you to look for particular features in his development; as each new one appears, take every opportunity to encourage him to exercise it. Treat him like a real person, not a toy, so that he can respond to you; and, above all, enjoy him! Never underestimate your own special, intimate knowledge of your own baby: you will know his patterns and reactions, likes and dislikes, fears and pleasures, sooner than anyone else.

Easy breastfeeding—postnatal advice

Yes, breastfeeding can be easy and enjoyable. An understanding of how breasts make milk and how your baby gets it will go a long way towards achieving this. A diagram of a lactating breast (producing milk) will help explain the terms used in this section.

The size of your breasts has little if any bearing on the amount of milk you make. This is under the control of hormones, helped by a good blood supply and diet. There are two main hormones involved. One, prolactin, is responsible for the amount of milk made. It is released into your bloodstream while your baby is feeding, so the more he feeds the more prolactin is produced, ensuring a good supply of milk for the next feed. This is the principle of demand and supply, which is the basis of breastfeeding. The other hormone is oxytocin. This is also released when your baby feeds, but whereas prolactin makes milk, oxytocin makes it available by causing the milk-producing cells to contract, forcing the milk down the ducts and out of the nipple. This is called the let-down reflex and you will probably feel it working as your baby feeds. Often it works so strongly that the pleasant tingling feeling of your milk letting down

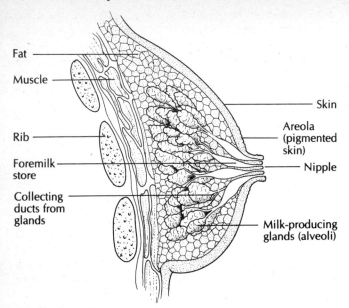

The breast, showing where milk is produced

becomes more like a 'full-to-bursting' feeling and you will
welcome your baby's eager feeding as it relieves this tension.

Your let-down reflex is what makes milk drip from side two
while you are feeding from side one. These drips can be
stopped by pressing on the nipple with your arm or you can
mop it up with a breast pad of some sort. Some mothers catch
this overflow in a sterilized shell and donate the milk to the
special care nursery of the local maternity unit, or freeze it for
their own baby's use when left with a baby-minder. Usually
your let-down reflex will work splendidly, but if you are
anxious, embarrassed, or rushed, the oxytocin won't be
released and your baby will get annoyed at having his milk
delayed. He will show this by pulling away from you and crying
angrily. You are going to have to keep calm, get comfortable,

relax, and smile! Your milk is there, and thinking about it is often enough to get it flowing.

One of the interesting facts about breast milk is that its composition changes as the feed progresses. At the start of each feed your baby will get foremilk, which is low in fat and calories and satisfies his thirst. As the let-down works, the richer hind-milk is produced which provides your baby with a high calorie, satisfying meal. This is probably what causes him to stop feeding from the first side but to recommence on side two, where he will get another drink followed by richer 'afters'. If feed times are restricted, the richer hind-milk is not taken and the baby does not settle after feeds and doesn't gain much weight despite having frequent, short feeds.

Most mothers want to know how often to feed their babies and for how long. This is a very personal matter between each mother and her baby and a pattern will gradually evolve that suits them. Feeding a baby is not just another job to be fitted into a neat timetable. It is the most important part of mothering, a time for being together, getting to know each other—a time for loving. Don't rush feed times: enjoy them.

As the composition of the breast milk and your baby's needs change, so feed times will vary. Here is the sort of pattern to expect, but please remember you and your baby are individuals: there can be infinite variations.

Colostrum, which your breasts have been making during pregnancy, is your baby's first food. It is a transition from placental feeding to milk and gently starts your baby's digestive system working. Although little in quantity, colostrum is high in quality and contains all the protein, minerals, fats, and vitamins that the baby needs. If your baby is allowed to have adequate feeds of colostrum, he may sleep for six to eight hours between feeds. This gives your nipples a chance to rest and recuperate, whereas limiting the feed time will allow your baby only an inadequate feed. He will either not settle or wake after a short time and need feeding again. After a few times of being removed from your breast before satisfying his appetite, he will try to feed more quickly and will grasp your nipple more tightly and so cause soreness. Do remember that babies have been around much longer than clocks and timed feeds are associated with bottle-feeding.

The birth of your baby triggers the production of the hormone prolactin and this induces the change from production of colostrum to production of milk, the change taking a day or two to complete. Your milk is perfectly suited to your baby. It looks thin and bluish and should not be compared either with formula milk or the 'doorstep' variety. However, as its protein and mineral content is lower than colostrum, it is digested more quickly and feeds become more frequent. Feed your baby when he wakens. He is not used to the feelings of hunger and will feel angry and alone if his needs are not met at once. He may ask to be fed as frequently as every hour and a half, and this is perfectly natural. By doing this, your milk supply is being built up and your baby learns that the world is a comforting place to be.

After a couple of hectic days and nights things will start to improve. Any engorgement (breasts feeling hot, swollen, and hard) will be subsiding and your milk supply is good. Your baby will start to go longer between feeds and will be having eight to ten feeds in twenty-four hours. The interval between feeds varies and this just underlines the fact that he has his own particular body rhythm and needs.

Night feeds are to be expected for some weeks yet, as your baby does not know the difference between night and day. Your milk supply is usually better during the night as prolactin levels are higher then. It may be easier to have your baby's crib right beside your bed, so that when he wakens for a feed it is a simple matter to bring him into bed with you and feed him. Don't worry if you doze off; your baby will be quite safe as long as neither you nor your partner have taken sleeping-pills or alcohol. Your baby will soon learn that night-times are for feeds only while daytimes are playtimes too.

How it's done

Your baby's instinct for survival and his search for food are very strong following a normal labour and delivery and as you hold him in your arms near your breast you will see him seeking for your nipple. Some babies like to nuzzle and lick the nipple or are content just to lie in mother's arms at this time, while others are keen to start feeding right away.

It is important that your baby gets on to your breast correctly from the beginning. Here are some points which may help.

1. Be in a comfortable position before starting to feed. There are no right or wrong ways and you will soon find what is best for you.

2. Use pillows to sit on if your stitches hurt, and on your lap to bring your baby to the breast if you are sitting on a chair or in

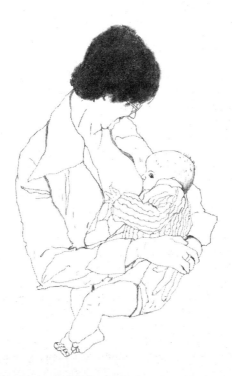

Sitting

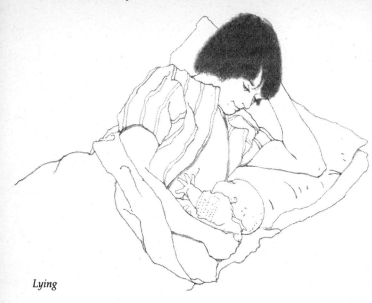

Lying

bed. You will get sore shoulders if you perch on the side of the bed bending over the baby. Rest your feet on the bed rail or inside your bed locker if your chair is too high.

3. Keep calm! Relax as much as possible using slow, relaxing breathing learned antenatally. Smile! Think milk!

4. Hold your baby so that he has to tilt his head back and touch your breast with his chin in order to get your nipple and areola into his mouth correctly. If you hold him too far towards your side he will have to put his chin on his chest to get your nipple into his mouth and that will hurt you.

5. When he is on correctly, you will see the top of his ear wiggling as he feeds. If his cheeks are going in and out as he sucks, he is not on properly. Break his suction by putting your little finger into the corner of his mouth, take him off and start again.

6. Support your breast from below, with the flat of your hand

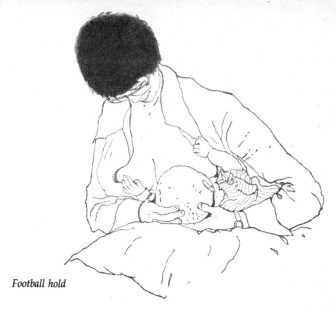

Football hold

against your rib-cage: this directs your milk down your baby's throat. Don't keep your finger on the top of your breast: this points the end of your nipple to your baby's hard palate where it will get bruised. It will also pull your nipple away from his mouth. Your baby will be able to breathe through the side of his nostril. If you can see part of his nostril, he can breathe.

Once your baby is on your breast he will feed in spurts. When he rests between sucking-spurts he will keep your nipple in his mouth. If you think he may have gone to sleep, a gentle jiggle will be sufficient to start him feeding again.

Usually there is no need to time feeds. Sore nipples are generally caused by incorrect feeding positions. Your baby will stop feeding when he has had enough, but if he goes on to 'comfort sucking'—chewing on the nipple and letting his cheeks balloon in and out—you can remove him from your breast, because this could make you very sore.

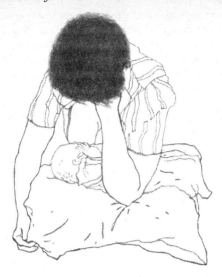

A position especially helpful when your ducts are blocked—sitting leaning forward over your baby, who is supported on a pillow on a low table, between your knees

A healthy, full-term baby, whose feed times are not restricted, does not need any complementary feeds, either of formula or sugar water. These will lessen his appetite for breast milk, causing him to go longer between feeds and so not stimulating your prolactin and therefore your milk supply. If your baby is not with you at night, a note pinned to his cot asking for him to be brought to you for feeding when he wakens will remind the night staff that you are breastfeeding.

If your baby is small-for-dates (smaller than expected given the dates by which you have been calculating), premature, jaundiced, or ill, your paediatrician will advise you accordingly.

Discomforts

Although breastfeeding should be easy and enjoyable, there are some discomforts at first for which you should be prepared.

Engorgement If you have been able to feed your baby as described, on demand, you will minimize the discomfort caused by early engorgement. This occurs between the second and fifth days usually. Your breasts feel hot, swollen, and hard. It is due to increased blood supply within the breast and the starting up of milk production. Extra fluid in the breast tissue is called oedema and you may have to ease it away from your nipple by gentle fingertip stroking so that the nipple can stand out for your baby. Also try:

- Cold compresses applied to your breasts straight after feeds. This will constrict the blood-vessels and let the oedema subside.

- Warm douching prior to feeds: helps to get your milk flowing.

- A latex nipple shield, if your nipple is still not protruding. Start the feed with it and remove it once your nipple has been drawn out.

- A firm, supporting bra. If you have a Mava bra you will probably need the long lace or the hooks let out to the maximum.

- Smoothing a little oil on your breasts, if they are still hard, and gently expressing some milk with a syringe-type breast pump. Avoid vigorous hand expressing as this can bruise the swollen tissues.

- Asking your midwife for some pain-killers, if you are in a lot of discomfort. Engorgement is only a temporary condition and is a sign that your breasts are working as expected.

Preventing sore nipples Nipple sensitivity increases during the first week after the baby is born and then subsides. The nipples feel very tender and you won't want to touch them. The area on the areola where your baby's gums go may feel bruised. This feeling can last for a few weeks, but is only uncomfortable at the start of feeds. To prevent your nipples getting bruised or cracked, here are some guide-lines:

- Follow the instructions (pp. 173–5) for getting your baby on to your breast correctly.

- There is no need to wash your breasts before or after each feed. Your daily bath is quite sufficient. Excessive washing removes the natural oils and predisposes to soggy, easily damaged skin.

- Change your feeding position frequently so that the pressure from your baby's gums is on a different part of the areola. Think of your breast as a clock-face and feed at 12, 3, 6, and 9 o'clock.

- Start feeds on alternate sides. A safety-pin on your bra strap will remind you with which side to start.

- Don't let the baby chew on your nipples or use them like a dummy.

- Let your nipples dry naturally at the end of each feed. A hairdrier is a comforting way to dry them. A drop of expressed milk allowed to dry on the nipple may help to prevent soreness.

- Many mothers do not use creams or sprays at all. If you do need to, use them sparingly. Always test for sensitivity first by putting a little in the flexure of your elbow. If there is no soreness or redness after an hour or two, you should be all right. Cream which has to be washed off your bra is wasted. Products which are specifically for nipples are not harmful to babies and need not be washed off before feeds. Creams containing steroids should be washed off.

- To keep your nipples dry between feeds use disposable breast pads, cut-up pieces of nappy roll, or clean cotton hankies. One-way nappies are excellent for keeping your skin dry as long as the backing material is not soaked. Tissues and toilet-paper tend to disintegrate and will lead to your spending a lot of time removing damp balls of paper from your breasts before feeds. Don't use drip-catching shells between feeds; they will make you leak more.

After pains   The oxytocin that is letting down your milk also makes your uterus contract. This is to get it back to its pre-

pregnancy size as quickly as possible. Unfortunately the contractions may be uncomfortable and tend to get worse with each baby. Remember your relaxation techniques and that smiling helps you to relax. If the contractions are upsetting your feed times, ask your midwife for some pain-killers a few minutes before you think you will be starting the feed. Difficult, but not impossible!

Enough milk?   You can be sure your baby is getting enough milk if:

- He settles contentedly after feeds. Remember the length of time he sleeps between feeds is not so important. He may feed two-hourly and then sleep five or six hours between the next feeds.
- He has a steady weight gain; 170 gm (6 oz) per week is average. Some babies put on 400 gm (14 oz), others 85 gm (3 oz) per week.
- His motions are soft and yellow. Breastfed babies are never constipated, although some open their bowels only once every five, seven, or even nine days. Others do it every feed.
- He has at least six wet nappies a day while not having any extra fluids.
- He looks happy and contented and his body feels firm and rounded.

How to maintain a good milk supply

1. Unrestricted feed times.

2. Eat well. Now is the time to eat for two. You will need 500 extra calories per day which can be taken in whatever form you like. Don't skip meals but try to have a snack and a drink at each feed time. Beware of going for many hours overnight without food while doing five or six feeds. Breastfeeding uses up 800–1,000 calories per day, so you will be using up your fat stores which were laid down during pregnancy particularly for this purpose.

3. Drink only to satisfy your thirst. Forcing yourself to take

more liquid than you want won't help. You don't have to drink milk to make milk. Go easy on the alcohol, although a glass of wine or beer can be an aid to relaxation.

4. Avoid drugs and smoking. Everything you eat goes through to your milk in some measure. If you do have to take medicines, remind your doctor that you are breastfeeding.

By demand feeding your baby your breasts soon produce the amount of milk that he requires. Don't feel threatened by 'demand' feeding. It can work both ways and once you are confident of your supply you can start making some demands yourself. You may need to waken your baby to feed him prior to going out or you may have to do half a feed now and the other half later. You can make this up to him by meeting his sucking demands later on when you have more time.

Many babies feed frequently in the late afternoon and evening. It may help if you prepare your evening meal early in the day so you do not have so many demands on your time later. Carrying your baby in a sling will allow you to get on with your work.

Mothers who have a more than adequate supply may find that their babies take too much milk but are still needing to satisfy their sucking urge. These babies bring back the excess milk and are fretful. A dummy could be the answer, or he may be quite happy to suck someone's little finger—perhaps Daddy's.

Father's support   And where does the father fit into all this? His role is a supportive one: to tell you what a great job you are doing and to top you up emotionally when you feel drained. It is the emotional part of parenting which is so demanding but is so difficult to prepare for and so hard to describe.

Your partner will be a buffer between you and your baby and the outside world. He can see when things are getting on top of you and can protect you from too many visitors.

On a practical level he can bring home take-away meals and help with any older children in the evening.

There are lots of ways he can share in the baby's care—it isn't just a matter of nappy-changing and bathing. Dads are good at calming small babies—perhaps the absence of the smell of milk persuades the baby to go to sleep. And the slightly older baby enjoys a boisterous game before bedtime—perhaps bathing will calm him down for sleep after the playtime.

Sex The desire for sexual intercourse comes from your hormones and some women feel particularly sexy whilst lactating. If your breasts are full, you will probably find it more comfortable to feed your baby first. This will also minimize the amount of milk which leaks at orgasm.

Although your periods may not return while you are fully breastfeeding, you still need to take contraceptive precautions, as ovulation occurs before the period. Your GP or Family Planning Clinic will discuss the various methods with you and your partner.

Conflicting advice This you will get plenty of! Remember that you and your baby are unique. What worked for everyone else may not be right for you. There are no hard and fast rules for breastfeeding. Try things. If they don't work, don't despair; try something else. Contact an NCT breastfeeding counsellor; she will help you to find out what is best for you and your baby. With new babies situations change frequently and so what is right today may not work tomorrow. Learn to be flexible and ignore advice you don't need.

Breastfeeding—coping with possible problems

Prevention of problems is better than trying to cure them. We hope you will have read our 'Easy breastfeeding' section in good time. Sometimes, however, there are difficulties and this section is to help you recognize and treat them.

Sore nipples

Prevention is discussed on pp. 177–8. Read the suggestions there again, checking your position and that your baby is properly on the breast. Then try some of the following suggestions.

1. Get really comfortable before starting to feed. Try to relax, remembering your antenatal classes; listen to some music; have a hot drink ready; have a warm bath.

2. Get the milk flowing before putting the baby to your breast. Thinking about milk helps the let-down reflex.

3. Feed your baby before he becomes ravenously hungry, wakening him if necessary and starting on the least sore side first as sucking is most vigorous at the start of a feed.

4. Expose your nipples to the air as much as possible, especially after feeds.

5. Wear plastic tea-strainers, with the handles cut off, over your nipples. These allow the air to circulate. Wash them at least once a day and do not wear them at night in case they put undue pressure on a duct.

6. Sit with nipples uncovered one foot away from a 40 watt light bulb for a few minutes four or five times a day.

7. Use a latex nipple shield, but remember that your baby will not get all your milk while feeding with it, so feeds will take longer and be more frequent.

8. If you are using cream or spray, stop. It may be the cause of the problem. A few people are allergic to some of these products.

9. If you have not been using any cream, you may find one useful. Get advice from your midwife, health visitor, or NCT breastfeeding counsellor. Vitamin E oil or calendula cream are natural products containing no chemicals which will speed healing if used sparingly and do not need to be washed off before a feed.

10. Stop wearing bra and breast pads at night. This may be messy but allows the skin to dry out.

11. Try shorter, more frequent feeds. This needs co-operation from junior!

12. If your baby has thrush in his mouth (white patches which won't rub off), or on his bottom (red, spotty rash), you may well have it on your nipples although you won't see anything. Your doctor can prescribe an appropriate remedy —homoeopathy can help here too.

Cracked nipples

Sometimes the skin of the nipple develops a crack, possibly due to incorrect feeding position. Cracks are very painful, particularly at the start of feeds, but they can heal very quickly. Here are some things you can do to prevent and help to heal cracked nipples.

1. Follow all the advice given for sore nipples.

2. Feed your baby on demand. He will then treat your nipples more gently as he is not angered and frustrated by timed, scheduled feeds. Remember, babies were around long before clocks.

3. Check and change your feeding position as on p. 178 (preventing sore nipples) *or*, if feeding is too painful, feed from the other side and hand express from the affected side. Generally hand or electric pumps aggravate a crack, but some mothers find them satisfactory. Give the expressed milk either from a spoon or a bottle. If your baby refuses the bottle, try using a specially designed teat which is more like a human nipple.

4. When the crack has healed, offer that breast second and restrict the feed time while the nipple remains tender.

5. Restrict comfort sucking on the sore side. Let the baby suck your finger or a dummy instead.

6. Vitamin E oil, gently applied, aids healing.

Other breast problems

Let's start with the most uncommon problem.

Breast abscess This can develop without warning, or it may follow on from a blocked duct or mastitis. It appears as a soft, painless swelling anywhere in the breast. If it is deep within the breast, the first sign may be pus mixed with the milk. You must see your doctor as soon as possible for antibiotics and probably to have the abscess incised and drained. It is not necessary to stop breastfeeding. Feed from the unaffected side; express from the affected side and discard the milk while there is pus or blood in it. Complementary formula feeds may be needed at this time. Natural yoghurt and/or complete vitamin B formula will help you to counteract the side-effects of antibiotics.

Engorgement   This may occur between the second and fifth days when your milk 'comes in'. See p. 177.

Using a latex nipple shield (which is worn over the nipple) will give your baby something to latch on to. His sucking then draws your nipple out. Once your milk is flowing you can remove the shield as your baby will not get all the milk that is available if you use it for the whole feed.

Should you have used the shield for some days and find that your baby refuses to go directly on to your breast, wean him off it by gradually cutting away more and more of the tip of the shield so that eventually he is on your breast with just a rim of rubber round it. Then you can abandon what remains of the shield.

Any pumps, shells, or shields must be washed after each use and sterilized. Cold-water chemical sterilization is the most convenient, effective method. You should prepare a fresh solution daily. Boiling briskly for five minutes is an alternative, especially for latex products.

Blocked ducts/mastitis   Occasionally one of the milk ducts may become blocked due to pressure from clothing or your hand during feeds, or overdistended due to rushed or missed feeds. A red, tender patch may be seen on the breast and there may be an underlying lump. You should get the milk flowing as soon as possible.

1. Do not give up breastfeeding; that will make the problem worse.

2. Feed frequently, particularly from the sore side.

3. Change baby's feeding position so that he clears all the

ducts. While feeding, lean forwards so that gravity will help to drain the breast (see illustration on p. 276).

4. A bath, shower, or warm flannels applied to the breast will help the milk to flow.

5. After feeds, gently massage any lumps towards the nipple. Combing the breast with a fine-toothed comb and soapy lather is a good way to do this.

6. Express as much milk as possible from the affected area by hand or breast pump.

7. Vigorous arm swinging exercises, or floor- or window-cleaning, can help by increasing the blood supply to the breast.

8. If there is no improvement in a few hours, see your doctor as mastitis could develop. He will probably prescribe antibiotics as a preventive measure. These will not harm your baby but do remind him that you are breastfeeding. You should not stop breastfeeding; your milk is not infected. The antibiotics may give your baby diarrhoea so he will want to feed more frequently. You should take natural yoghurt and/or complete vitamin B formula to counteract the side-effects of the antibiotics.

If you do develop mastitis you will feel that you are getting the flu. The hot, shivery, achy feelings are due to milk which has leaked into the breast tissue. Do not stop feeding your baby; he is your best ally right now! Also, you should:

1. Rest—in bed preferably. Get someone to help with shopping and other children.

2. Take plenty of fluids while you are feverish.

3. Apply hot or cold compresses to the affected area, whichever is most comforting.

You will feel better as soon as you get the milk flowing and the breast emptied. Then try to find out what caused the trouble.

Remember what the first feelings were like. If you feel that a blocked duct may be occurring again, express your milk and change your feeding position: you may be able to avert an attack.

Stopping breastfeeding   If you don't start breastfeeding or you change to bottle-feeding in the first week, your breasts will continue to make milk for a few days. You will experience engorgement, which you can treat with cold compresses and by wearing a firm bra. Some midwives advise expressing once with an electric pump, but not more often as you will increase the milk supply. Any expressed milk can be offered to the tiny babies in the special care nursery.

After lactation   Whenever you stop lactating, be it after days, months, or years, it takes some time for the milk glands to stop working. When you are stopping breastfeeding it is best to wean slowly to cause least discomfort to yourself. After the milk glands have stopped producing milk the breast feels and looks empty. Don't be anxious, gradually fat will be laid down in your breasts and your figure will be restored.

If you have read straight through this section, you may wonder why anyone breastfeeds at all if these problems can occur! In fact many mothers feed without any problems at all. Some experience one or two at some time, but no one gets all the problems at once.

Remember the emphasis is on avoidance and quick first aid. If at any time you are in doubt and want to talk about feeding, contact your NCT breastfeeding counsellor, who is trained to listen and to give non-medical information which will help you decide what to do.

How to express and store breast milk

There is no need to express milk in the ordinary course of breastfeeding, but you may need to collect and/or store milk in some special circumstances, for example:

- If your baby is in hospital or cannot suck, and you want to collect all your milk to be given to him by bottle or tube.
- If you are going to be temporarily away from your baby and

you want to save up milk for one or more bottles while you are away.

- If your doctor or midwife advises it, to relieve engorged breasts and to help the baby get a better position on the nipple.
- If your nipples are cracked and you have to rest them (hand expressing only please, as pumps can be too harsh).
- If you are breastfeeding your own baby, and also want to donate milk to a milk bank for premature and sick babies.

The method of collection you choose, and how often you do it, will depend on your particular circumstances.

Collecting drip-milk The simplest method, if you are feeding your own baby, is to catch drips from one breast while the baby feeds from the other. This way the baby does all the work, and some mothers manage to produce quite large amounts, especially in the early weeks of breastfeeding. The milk can be collected in any sterile container, plastic or glass, or a specially designed 'drip-catcher' or shell. If you are collecting milk for a hospital milk bank, the hospital will probably provide containers for the milk.

'Drip-milk' is usually mixed with other expressed breast milk if used in hospital as it is mainly foremilk, which is low in fat.

Hand expressing Hand expressing requires no special equipment and is inexpensive. However, not everyone finds it easy to acquire the knack and, as it is not always efficient at emptying the breast, it is probably most useful if you have to express only a small amount, or for a short period (for example if you become very engorged or if your nipples are cracked). The best way to learn is from a midwife or a breastfeeding mother—*before* the birth of your baby so you will know how to do it even though it may not be necessary. Don't be discouraged, or squeeze so hard that you hurt yourself, if you can only squeeze a few drops at the beginning; you can become very efficient at it with a little practice.

The breast is made up of fifteen to twenty segments. Each

segment contains milk-producing cells connected to the nipple by a system of ducts. Before each duct opens on to the nipple, it enlarges to form a reservoir. It is over these reservoirs that pressure needs to be applied when expressing milk. They are located where the darker skin of the areola merges into the 'normal' skin of the breast. See illustration on p. 170.

When hand expressing, try to choose a time when you are not rushed. Wash your hands and dry them on a clean towel and make yourself comfortable before you start. Thinking about the baby and milk helps the let-down reflex to work. So does relaxation—remember the breathing that you learnt at ante-natal classes. Listening to music can also help.

To encourage the milk to flow down the ducts apply hot compresses before starting to express, and stroke the breast very gently, in the direction of the nipple, with a delicate fingertip touch before and during expressing.

You will probably find it easier to express the left breast with the right hand and vice versa.

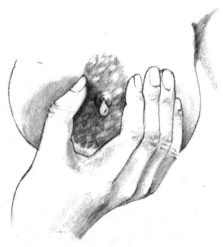

Expressing milk

Support your left breast with your right hand and squeeze the milk sacs beneath the areola between your thumb and your hand. Press your thumb and hand into the breast towards your rib-cage, then squeeze them rhythmically together. The pressure needs to be very firm to get the first few drops of milk. Your fingers should not slide over the skin of the areola or touch the nipple.

Move your hand around the areola to make sure that all the sacs are emptied.

Other means of helping to get the let-down reflex going are, for example, gently stimulating the nipple, or massaging the breast with warm water (or even using the baby if he is willing). Once the milk is flowing, expression is easier.

Change hands and breasts frequently to give your tired muscles a rest—they will become used to expressing with practice—and to let the sacs refill with more milk.

Hand pumps　If you have to express your milk regularly for a babysitter to give in a bottle, a hand pump is useful. There are two main types on the market.

(a) A pump which works on the syringe principle. By working the outer cylinder in and out, suction is built up and milk is expressed. The expressed milk collects in the inner cylinder, which holds about 9 ml or 3 fl oz and doubles as a feeding-bottle.

(b) What is sometimes called a 'breast reliever'. This consists of a glass cylinder, having one end flared to fit over the nipple and areola, the other end fitted with a plastic bulb, and a reservoir in the middle (which holds up to 57 ml (2 fl oz)). By squeezing and releasing the bulb, milk is expressed from the breast. It can be used on one side while the baby feeds from the other. Squeeze as gently as possible until you get used to the action.

Hand pumps are best sterilized using cold-water sterilizing solution. Separate the parts and ensure that all pieces are full of solution and submerged.

Electric pumps　If you have a premature or sick baby you could consider using an electric breast pump. These work by applying a rhythmical suction to the nipple and areola. They are efficient at obtaining the milk and sometimes help to improve the shape of flat nipples. Many maternity units have electric pumps. In some areas these pumps can be hired out from the NCT for home use. Their action is carefully designed to avoid damage to the nipple. The milk collects in a beaker which is used by one mother only, to avoid the risk of cross infection. Details of how to use the electric pump may be found in the manufacturer's instruction leaflet. If you use some hiring scheme other than the NCT's national scheme and are provided with a glass beaker, be scrupulous about sterilizing it.

When to express

A good time is after a relaxing bath or shower. It is difficult to express milk if you are in a rush. If you are expressing all your milk for your own baby in hospital you will need to express at least six times a day in order to maintain your milk supply. If you need to increase your supply, try expressing more often and use a pump.

If you are breastfeeding your own baby and only want to express the occasional feed for later use (for example if you are going out), try expressing a couple of hours after the baby has had a good feed—the breasts will have refilled again by the time he wants another feed. Many mothers find they have most milk in the morning. When the baby drops a night feed, last thing at night is a good time to express.

Great care must be taken if you are expressing engorged breasts—it is very easy to bruise the tissues of the breast. It is usually only necessary to express enough milk to soften the areola, so that the baby can 'get on'.

Hygiene

Germs multiply rapidly in milk so it is important to avoid introducing any into it.

Always wash your hands before collecting milk and dry them on a clean towel kept especially for this purpose.

Wash containers etc. in hot, soapy water to remove the milk film. Soak them in cold water if you cannot wash them immediately after use.

If the milk is to be used at home, or if it is to be taken to hospital, all the utensils should be sterilized in a cold-water sterilizing solution (which must be changed daily), or by boiling briskly for five minutes. Do not put any metal parts in the sterilizing solution.

Storage

1. Containers for home use might be plastic freezer containers, feeding-bottles which can be boiled or frozen without damage, or sterile plastic bags. They must be sealed.

Hospitals supply pre-sterilized bottles, but if these are to be kept for several days before filling, it is a good idea to keep them in the sterilizing solution too. Rinse in boiled water before use.

2. Label each container with the date of collection (and your name, if it is going to hospital). If the container is in the ordinary part of the refrigerator you can top it up with more milk collected the same day.

3. Breast milk will keep for twenty-four hours in the ordinary part of the refrigerator, or it can be deep-frozen and kept up to six months. If you are donating to a milk bank check with your hospital for their specific requirements for the length of time milk can be kept. Some prefer to use the milk untreated and in this case the 'fresher' it is, the better. Chill the milk as quickly as possible. Stand the container in cold running water if you do not have a fridge.

4. If you are taking milk to hospital every day and have no fridge, you can store it overnight in an insulated container with an ice-pack (available from camping shops). The container can be a thickly padded bag or of polystyrene or cardboard lined thickly with newspaper. Leave as little airspace around the bottles as possible, and keep the ice-pack on top of the bottles with an insulated lid over the top. Keep the container in the coldest, draughtiest place you can. The hospital could be freezing one ice-pack for you while you are using another. This

method is also useful if you have to leave milk out for collection and when it is being transported.

5. When you want to use frozen EBM (expressed breast milk), defrost it as quickly as possible by standing the container in hot water.

Milk banks

Before you donate milk to a milk bank, check with the hospital to see what conditions they make. Special precautions have to be taken when babies are very weak and the milk comes from a donor. They may not accept your milk if you smoke, take the contraceptive pill, or other drugs. Some hospitals will not take milk that has been frozen as they cannot be sure the temperature has been constant. Report to the hospital if you have been in contact with an infectious disease, although this won't necessarily mean that you have to stop donating, and also if you have developed anything wrong with you.

For very tiny babies who weigh less than 1.5 kg (3¼ lb) some paediatricians prefer to add extra nutrients to mother's EBM or to use specialized high-protein formula feed. If this happens to you, express your milk regularly and store it in a freezer ready for the day when your baby is big enough to have it. You will then have your own milk to draw on if necessary.

Bottle-feeding

Bottle-feeding is an alternative to breastfeeding, when breast-feeding is not possible through illness, lack of help, choice, or the few medical conditions which contra-indicate breastfeed-ing. It is used occasionally to complement breastfeeding.

The aims are the same, whatever method of feeding is used: to promote the bond between mother and baby, and to provide the best available nutrition. With any new baby, the senses of hearing, touch, and smell are more developed than sight, so that skin contact and warmth play a part in feeding, as does talking to the baby. Feeding time is a special time in which to learn to know and love each other.

Bottle-feeding has been known through the ages, but it is only in the last fifty years that it has become safe enough to be widely used. Further safety measures have been introduced in this country in recent years.

Bottle-feeding generally means using cows' milk or a modification of cows' milk. Soya bean substitutes can be prescribed for babies who have an allergy to cows' milk, and modified goats' milk is also used occasionally. There are also completely synthetic products available for babies with allergies to all of these formulas.

Milk is a complete food, a fluid containing protein, sugar, salts, fats, and some vitamins, and each species of mammal provides a milk which is uniquely suited to its own young. To adapt cows' milk for human babies, careful scientific modification is necessary to bring it closer to human milk, although there are still many differences.

Instructions for preparing feeds vary with each manufacturer and are clearly indicated on each packet. These must be followed carefully, if a safe and correct formula is to be achieved.

Bottle-feeding is more cumbersome than breastfeeding, but it is not necessarily more difficult and can be carried out as tenderly, providing much pleasure for the baby.

Points to remember

Adequate sterilization is vital: cold-water sterilization of all equipment using a hypochlorite solution is simple and generally preferable, but brisk boiling for a minimum of five minutes can be equally effective. All items must be submerged. Any sterilizing agent should be rinsed off pumps, bottles, etc. with recently boiled water just before use. Yesterday's sterilizing solution can be used to disinfect dishcloths or wipe down work surfaces.

A modified milk suitable for infants under six months should be chosen for your new baby. Check with the midwife or health visitor for a suitable brand.

Prepare each feed as instructed, using only the measuring scoop provided. *Do not* overfill the scoop, compress the powder in it, or add additional scoops.

Do not store prepared feeds, except covered in a refrigerator, and then for no longer than 24 hours. If travelling, do not carry warm feeds, for instance, in thermos flasks, because bacteria multiply rapidly in warm milk. Keep it cold (perhaps with a freezing pack) and then warm it immediately before feeding.

Modern modified milks are safer than the older brands in common use until quite recently, but do not satisfy a baby for the 'routine' four hours. The pattern is more like breastfeeding, with varying amounts of feed being taken and at varying intervals.

Remember that babies are often thirsty and not always hungry. As a basic guide-line, the baby may need feeding between three- and five-hourly at first. If he wants a feed sooner than three-hourly you could offer extra water or add 15–30 ml ($\frac{1}{2}$–1 fl oz) of extra water to the feed. Your baby may not be able to cope with the manufacturer's recommended strength of feed and if he possets a lot (brings back small quanties of milk after feeds) the feed can be made weaker by adding 30 ml (1 fl oz) of extra water *or* by omitting one scoop of the formula. Talk about this with your health visitor or doctor, to make sure that your baby is receiving adequate nutrition.

Modified milks contain essential vitamins. Extra vitamins are unnecessary and extra vitamins A and D can be harmful.

Feeds may be given cold, warm, or at room temperature, but must never be given hot. Test the milk by running a few drops on the inside of your wrist. It should feel neither warm nor cold. A bottle should not be re-heated, and left-over formula should be thrown away.

There are variations in shapes of teats and in sizes of holes. A medium-holed teat is the usual choice, but continual steriliza- tion does alter the size of the hole. Check daily, especially if the baby tires easily during feeding. Feeds normally take between ten and forty minutes.

It is usual for young babies to swallow air when feeding and it is advisable to stop once or twice to allow the baby to burp. This can be achieved by sitting the baby up and gently rocking him or rubbing his back. Do not hold him completely upright, but rather, sloping slightly backwards supported by your arm. The teat needs to be released frequently to let air enter the bottle.

Clean the bottles with a bottle-brush—first with cold water, immediately after feeding, to remove the protein film—then with hot soapy water to remove the fat. Rub the teats with salt, inside and out. Return everything to the chemical sterilizing solution, which should be made up daily. Always rinse again with cooled boiled water before use.

Remember to talk to and cuddle your baby during feeding times and never leave him alone with a bottle, even for a moment, in case he chokes.

You must continue to sterilize your baby's bottles for as long as milk is offered in them.

Early days

Your baby may be sleepy at times at first. This will improve as he gets older. Bowel movements alter in the early days, and bottle-fed babies are sometimes slightly constipated. Extra water helps, but if it is a problem, ask your health visitor for advice. There are homoeopathic remedies which have been found helpful for treating colicky babies.

New babies need time and energy spent on them, and you may well be tired. Eat sensibly and rest when you can; you will feel better for it.

Introducing solid foods

During the first four months, a diet of milk and, in some cases, a vitamin supplement, is all that is required to ensure an alert and contented baby with a healthy weight gain of 113–200 g (4–7 oz) per week, which should taper off to about 450 g (1 lb) a month by the seventh month. After the fourth month, little tastes of puréed foods can be offered in order to pave the way for a more varied diet at approximately six months.

If your baby is over four months old, and, despite more frequent milk feeds, seems interested in more, this will probably mean readiness for solid food. If you are breastfeeding, you judge by the baby's demands; if you are bottle-feeding, the baby may be taking 1 litre (30–35 fl oz) of milk a day when he starts to want solids.

Start with very small quantities—about a teaspoonful—and do not make a great fuss about the procedure. It does not matter, from a nutritional point of view, if the baby does not eat the food. Do not interpret any rejection of the food as a rejection of you.

Starting mixed feeding

Usually the 2 p.m. or lunchtime feed is a good one at which to start solids. If you are breastfeeding, offer the breast before the solids to maintain your milk supply. Later, one breast can be offered, then the solids, and then the other breast. This ensures that at least one breast is emptied at each feed. If you are bottle-feeding, start by giving most of the milk first, then the solid food, slowly decreasing the amount of milk offered as the amount of solid food is increased. As your baby becomes more interested in solid foods, he may prefer them first and his milk at the end of the meal.

Vegetables and fruit make a better introduction than cereal. At first purée or sieve the food to a smooth, semi-liquid consistency. A manual food blender is best for small amounts: larger amounts can be prepared in an electric blender if you have one. Your baby will suck at the spoon to begin with and perhaps spit the spoonful out simply because he is not used to dealing with food in this form, but he should soon acquire the new skill. If he rejects it absolutely, leave it for a few days and try again. This may happen several times. Home-made purée will keep in the fridge for up to 48 hours, or can be deep-frozen in plastic ice-cube trays.

Quantities

No more than one teaspoonful should be offered the first time. Increase amounts very slowly so that after two to three months the baby is having a first course of protein (such as beans, cheese, meat, or fish) with vegetables and a second course of pudding or fruit—about 100–150 g (4–6 oz) in all— with a drink of juice or water afterwards. If the baby is uncomfortable, colicky, or has unusual bowel motions, you are probably going too fast. When one food is accepted, add another, gradually increasing the variety. Babies can take time to get used to savoury foods, so concentrate on bland vegetables such as carrot, potatoes, and cauliflower first.

Dos

In a family with a history of allergies, consult your doctor about which foods to delay introducing, usually eggs, wheat, and cows' milk.

Introduce each new food individually, so that foods which disagree with the baby may be readily identified. Sieve or purée foods very carefully in the beginning, progressing to mashing with a fork at about six or seven months. Offer juice or water by cup at about five months; try again a week later if it is rejected.

As soon as your baby can hold a spoon, offer him one while you are feeding him and encourage him to scoop up some of his own dinner. Guide his hand to get the food into his mouth. Do not be dismayed if he throws it on the floor; put a plastic sheet or cloth under the high chair.

Include the baby in family meals at least once a day when solids have been established, to encourage the child's enjoyment of his food and imitation of others at the table.

When your baby is having a full lunch or dinner of first and second courses, offer diluted fruit juice (not squash) or plain boiled water afterwards instead of the breast or bottle feed.

If the baby is ready, start small amounts of solid food at breakfast or tea when he is six or seven months old. If you progress at this rate, he will probably be having three meals a day, mainly from the family menu, by nine to twelve months of age. Continue with milk at breakfast and tea, also at bedtime if required. All babies will differ, so this should only be a general guide.

Don'ts

Do not offer new solids to a baby crying with hunger; this will annoy him and colour his opinion of solid food. Do not transmit your own likes and dislikes. Your voice, tone, and facial expressions tell all!

Never re-use a tin or jar of food into which you have dipped the eating spoon. The saliva on the spoon will start a breakdown of the food causing it to decay rapidly. At the start of the meal, using a clean spoon, spoon the amount you require into a dish. Do not reheat food left over from the baby's meal.

Avoid the use of sweets. Remember that a 'sweet tooth' is developed, not inherited, and do not automatically sweeten foods. Babies over a year old can have raisins instead of sweets. Most fruits, drinks, and cereals are tolerated without sugar.

Do not add salt to a baby's food.

If you are bottle-feeding, do not add cereal to the milk as this may prevent the calcium in the milk being used effectively.

Do not leave a young baby of six months alone with food on which he may choke or gag.

First foods

Fruits are ideal beginners. Puréed and sieved apples, pears, and ripe bananas can be prepared in amounts to last several days and stored in a clean container in the fridge or freezer in covered plastic ice-cube trays. When the baby can chew (around six to eight months), he can be given very thinly sliced raw apple or pear to hold and chew. Watch and see that he doesn't choke on it.

Vegetables   Virtually any puréed vegetables can be served. Skinned, puréed tomato is particularly convenient. After the first year, well-washed and scrubbed vegetables can be given raw, for example carrot sticks.

The best way to cook fruits and vegetables is to put just enough water into a saucepan to cover the bottom. While the water is boiling, drop in the finely chopped fruit or vegetables, bring back to the boil rapidly and reduce the heat to simmer. Cook for the minimum time possible; do not add salt to the vegetables.

Meats These foods are fibrous and so must be cooked very well and blended thoroughly. Add some of the meat juices, broth, or water to moisten. Use any lean meat that you eat. Avoid meat which has been ground by the butcher as the surfaces have been handled and they are usually high in fat and fibre content. You can, of course, mince your own meat. At eight to ten months, meat can be offered minced and the baby can chew on a defatted and meaty cooked bone which has no sharp edges or splinters.

Fish White fish may be introduced cautiously after six months, but leave oily fish such as sardines, herring, or mackerel until the second year, and do not give a baby salted or smoked fish such as kippers or smoked haddock. When it is fully cooked the fish will separate easily into flakes; if cooking fillets or cutlets a white curd-like substance will form between the flakes indicating that the fish is cooked. Be careful to remove all bones.

Vegetarian food Instead of meat and fish, vegetarians can offer 'soya meats' (those which do not contain monosodium glutamate), lentil and nut roasts and mixed vegetable proteins suitably puréed. (Suggestions for vegetarian menus can be had from the Vegetarian Society.)

Eggs After six months, begin using the yolk only, raw or cooked, sieved and stirred into fruit or vegetable purées. Do not introduce the white of the egg until you are sure that the yolk is tolerated.

Cheese Any mild, finely grated hard cheese can be given, perhaps added to a white sauce and cooked to a smooth paste.

Cottage and cream cheese can also be sieved with the baby's food. Melted cheese should not be given to a baby as it becomes stringy and indigestible.

Breads and cereals Cereals should never be the predominant part of a meal. Introduce rice, oats, or barley cereal first and delay the use of wheat cereal as some babies may be allergic to the gluten in wheat. At about seven months, toasted bread or rusks are excellent finger foods and teething aids, but the baby needs to be watched while eating them to see that he doesn't choke.

Milk and milk puddings Introduce small amounts of cows' milk after the sixth month, in a cup, at mealtimes. To be on the safe side this should be scalded and diluted until the baby is one year old. Milk puddings, custards, or junkets can be served as a second course with fruit. Yoghurt too can be included if the baby likes it. Do not force cows' milk on your child if he does not like it.

Tins and jars of baby foods These are useful for convenience (though expensive), but read the label carefully before buying. The contents are listed in order of their quantities, largest amounts first. Avoid those containing large amounts of cereal, wheat starch, or sugar.

A balanced diet

Adults and children should eat some foods containing each of the following daily: proteins, vitamins, carbohydrates, fats (see p. 42). Babies should not have very spicy foods, fruit squashes, unripe fruit, fruit with many seeds, coffee, cream cakes, and processed cereals. They may, however, be given very weak tea.

Points to remember

Mealtimes should be happy, so don't force food on your child. Reintroduce any rejected foods without fuss at a later time. Always be ready to mark time if the baby is teething or off colour. Be guided by the baby's reaction: if he is not forced he will soon regain his appetite. Don't equate food with love: when he rejects your cooking, he is not rejecting *you*!

A hungry baby will be eager and interested; if he just plays with the food and tries to throw it around, he is probably not hungry enough. Give him less next time.

Encourage independence: a child should be allowed to feed himself as soon as he wants to try. From seven to nine months provide part of each meal chopped or sliced so that he can finger-feed himself.

Caring for the new baby— things you will need

Getting a household ready for a first baby can seem to involve an incredible number of details and preparations for all kinds of possibilities. Advice will come from everywhere—from family and friends as well as from babycare manufacturers—so you will need to plan which of the many possible additions to your equipment you will want. If you know that people may be wanting to give you something for the baby, you may find that a list of possibilities is helpful.

The basics are:

- *A place to sleep*
  Carry-cot, basket even a box or drawer with a suitable lining and mattress (if buying second-hand equipment make sure it is thoroughly cleaned, repainted, etc. before you use it for your baby)

  (eventually a pram and/or cot)

  Sheets—cut up old ones, or use a pillowcase with the mattress inside it

  Blankets/pram or cot covers/shawls (especially washable ones)

- *Clothes and a place to keep them*

    Nappies and pins

    Liners

    Plastic or waterproofed nylon pants with legs wide enough to let in plenty of air

    Babygrow suits or nightgowns

    Vests

    Cardigans

    Outdoor clothing according to season (e.g. for winter—hats, bootees, top-to-toe suit with a hood and feet, mittens)

- *A place to feed which is comfortable for you*

- *Laundering requisites*

    Buckets, preferably with lids, in which to soak used nappies

    Soaking/sterilizing solution

    Soap or detergent

- *Nappy-changing requisites and a place to change—warm; comfortable for you both*

    Something to remove bowel motions from skin (e.g. cotton wool/toilet roll/wet flannel)

    Spare nappy pins

- *Bath requisites and place to bath—warm; comfortable for you both*

    Baby bath/washing-up bowl/or kitchen sink

    Baby soap and shampoo

    Towels, flannels, sponge

Basic care of your new baby

Mothering and fathering are a matter of common sense and individual taste. There are few right or wrong ways to do things, just as there is no standard way of being a daughter, wife, son, or husband. You and your baby will establish a way of life which suits you all best; the fact that your methods may drive someone else crazy is immaterial. There are no 'musts' about nappy changing, bathing, doing the laundry, or dressing the baby: be as unsystematic or meticulous as you like. The baby will know only whether or not you are happy and confident in your handling of him—and that is all he will care about.

If you have any problems they are likely to be caused by lack of experience, and only time can rectify that. People do not expect to be able to type the moment they sit down in front of a typewriter, or to be able to drive the first time they find themselves at the wheel of a car. It is the same with parenthood—it takes time and practice. If this is your first baby, you may find the following guidelines helpful, but make your own variations and discoveries. Ask your parents, friends, and health visitor for advice too, but feel free to pick and choose what suits you from the abundance of advice you will be given!

Clothing

Babies do not care how they look. They just want to be warm and dry and they loathe being dressed and undressed. You will probably not need many first-size clothes, just vests, babygrow suits, or nightdresses and cardigans. As far as possible get things that open either all at the back or all at the front so that you need not turn the baby over more than once when dressing or undressing him. Avoid long strings and ribbons; they soon get sucked and chewed and can be dangerous. Mittens are best made in fabric rather than knitted, so that there are no loose loops in which little fingers can be caught, but both these and bonnets are only necessary in cold weather. A couple of soft shawls will envelop the baby snugly when carrying him from room to room—again avoid long fringes or knitted patterns with large holes. You can tell whether or not the baby is warm enough by feeling the skin under the back of his collar.

Changing nappies

Nappies seem to preoccupy everyone in discussing babycare. The point is to keep the baby reasonably clean and dry and not complicate the matter further. At first you may feel that it is all rather messy and unpleasant, but eventually even the most squeamish of people find they can deal quickly and efficiently with their own babies' excreta.

It is a false economy to skimp on the quality and quantity of the towelling nappies you may buy. Thick nappies do not need to be changed so frequently and should retain their absorbent texture. You will need about 1½ to 2½ dozen depending on your laundering and drying arrangements. At first, a new baby can use up to eight nappies a day. You may prefer to use disposable nappies although for some babies they are quite inadequate and the babies' skin becomes red and sore. You may be able to obtain fleeced cotton twill nappies, which are by far the softest.

There are three basic ways of putting on babies' towelling nappies and the proponents of each method swear by it as 'the only sensible way'! The three methods are illustrated below. Try them out and see which one suits your baby best.

Plastic pants come in various types. Avoid those with very tight elastic around the legs; they can cut into the baby's flesh and make nappy rash worse by preventing the circulation of air around the nappy inside. Tie-on pants make a neat 'parcel' of the nappy and allow air circulation without any constriction at the top of the legs. Pants which fasten with poppers at the sides and have padded leg-holes are also comfortable for the baby and can be obtained in appropriate sizes. Some babies can never wear plastic pants because their skins are too delicate. Two towelling nappies make an adequate substitute. In any case, you may wish to avoid plastic pants as far as possible for a very young baby—imagine your own body steaming under a tight plastic mackintosh 24 hours a day, seven days a week!

Throw-away nappy liners are very useful for disposing of your baby's bowel motions and will help prevent staining of towelling nappies. Some of the more expensive disposable

A. KITE SHAPE

1. Fold sides into centre as shown.
2. Fold top and bottom corners inwards, thus producing equal thickness everywhere.
3. Fold round baby's legs and pin at sides.

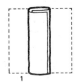

B. AMERICAN SHAPE

1. Fold nappy so that there are three thicknesses lengthwise (for a tiny baby fold into four so that the resulting strip is narrower).
2. Fold lower third up to make a thicker part to go at front or back, as required.
3. Simply place between baby's legs and pin at sides.

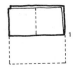 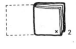

C. ORIENTAL SHAPE

1. Fold nappy in half upwards.
2. Fold in half again, left to right.
3. Draw top layer of nappy from top right corner over to the left, holding other layers down, so that corner 'x' (see stage 2) arrives at top left centre (see stage 3).
4. Reverse whole nappy face downwards.
5. Fold straight edge on left into the centre, leaving the triangular 'wing' behind.
6. Fold thick strip between baby's legs and pin to 'wings'.

liners can be soaked, washed, and re-used, assuming they have only been wet, not soiled. One-way fabric nappy liners are excellent for keeping your baby's bottom dry, but be careful not to clog the material with ointment or cream.

Have everything ready before you pick up the baby to change his nappy, so that you do not have to keep putting him down while you rush off to find something. It maddens him and will madden you.

If, for any reason, your baby develops nappy rash, expose his bottom to the air as much as possible (though this may involve lots of puddles, particularly with boys!) Try various proprietary ointments, or ask your doctor or health visitor's advice about available brands. Skin varies so much between individuals that a cream which will work wonders for one baby may have no effect at all on his siblings.

If your baby is taking antibiotics (or you are taking them and breastfeeding him) do not use zinc and castor-oil cream on his bottom as this itself may cause a rash. Do not use it either if your baby has thrush. It is wise not to use mineral-based baby oils on skin which is sore or broken. Baby lotion can be very astringent.

The world will not cave in around your ears if the baby's nappy is not changed at the middle-of-the-night feed. If he tends to produce a lot of urine which leaks into the cot overnight, try putting on two nappies: thick and thin towelling nappies, or a towelling nappy and a disposable one. A one-way nappy liner should ensure that the skin does not become sore.

The safest place for the baby to be when he is being changed is on the floor. He cannot fall anywhere!

Bathing

It is not necessary to bath a baby every day, so long as he is kept clean. Again, the matter can be made to seem unnecessarily complex. The main points to remember are: keep the baby warm; have everything ready in advance; wash his face and scalp first and his bottom later; and hold him firmly.

The usual way to bath a baby is in a special baby bath, but you can use a large washing-up bowl or a sink where the sharp taps have been covered by flannels. Before you bath the baby, wrap a large bath towel around your middle and have the room warm enough for you to bath him in a leisurely way. Check with your elbow or the inside of your wrist that the water is comfortably warm: babies don't like water too hot. Have everything ready to wash, dry and re-dress the baby before you undress him. Remember, you don't need much water, and as long as you wash his face and bottom the process need not be prolonged. Hold him on your lap and wash his face, then use a tiny amount of baby shampoo to wash his head thoroughly. Hold his head over the bath to rinse away the suds. Handling a slippery small baby for a bath is an art and at first feels very precarious. Lower him gently into the water, with the back of his head resting against your left wrist and your left finger and thumb grasped firmly around his left arm just below the armpit, and your right hand under his legs or bottom. Until you are experienced at this, simply hold him there, just swishing the water gently around him with your right hand. If he shows any fright, try holding his arms firmly against his chest and he will be reassured. Lift him out and wrap him quickly in a warm towel, and let him feel secure and enveloped in comfort before you pat him dry, and dress him.

It is not necessary to use soap or any other washing agent. The baby is not 'dirty' in the conventional sense of the word, so if you are worried about dropping him when he is slippery, just sponge him with the bath water. If you want to massage your baby before his bath, use a mild, pure baby soap. Baby bath-care liquids tend to be drying and unsuitable for some babies' skins.

The trickiest parts of a new baby to dry are the folds of skin under the arms and in the neck. Be careful, too, to dry in the groin and behind the ears. Avoid putting powder on wet patches; it just makes a 'pudding'.

There is no 'correct' time to bath a baby, the choice is yours. However it is not fair—on you or the baby—to give him a bath when he is very hungry, so do it between feeds when he is awake or, if it does not make him sick, after a feed. Some babies find baths very soothing and, if yours has a crying time, a warm luxurious bath may help to quiet him.

If your baby hates being bathed in the conventional way, you can try taking him into the ordinary bath with *you* (it may give you more confidence to have a non-slip mat on the bottom of the bath). Get in and out of the bath with the baby held firmly against your shoulder with one hand, and use the other to support yourself. Lie in the bath and sit him, or lie him, on your chest (or propped up, facing you, with his back supported against your raised thighs). Your presence and the reassuring nearness of your breasts should make the baby quite relaxed, and this mutual bathtime will be a happy and privately loving time for both of you. Keep the water comfortably warm but not too hot for the baby. Another way to calm an anxious baby is to bath him wrapped up in a towel. It also makes him less slippery.

Laundry

A small baby generates an incredible amount of washing. Since the turnover is rapid, it is essential to see that everything is adequately aired. Ironing, incidentally, is not one of the essentials in the life of a new baby, or of a new mother, and can safely be omitted.

If washing by hand see that things are well rinsed, and whether by hand or machine, do not use too much detergent or soap powder. If you use nappy-sterilizing solution (or diluted household bleach, or even washing soda) to soak nappies, they do not need boiling. Do not leave them in the solution too long, or it will smell revolting. Make up a fresh solution each day, and don't be tempted to use up yesterday's bottle sterilizing solution. That will still be effective for dishcloths or for washing down work surfaces, but is no longer able to cope with soiled nappies.

Sunshine will help to bleach nappies and rainwater softens them, so if you have enough it is a good idea to hang them out for a blow on the line whatever the weather. A tumbledrier is very useful for drying clothes and nappies or, if your home is centrally heated, the radiators will be useful too. White nappies hanging over white radiators do not look too obtrusive.

Fabric conditioner is best avoided altogether. It will of course help to keep the nappies soft, but it may cause an adverse reaction on your baby's skin. A compromise is to use the conditioner only occasionally and check for adverse reactions. It appears to coat the fibres and make them less absorbent.

Socializing

Some mothers are most attracted to their babies when they are very tiny, seeing them as wonderful complex little people who somehow encompass the wisdom of the ages together with an awesome 'newness'. They find their maternal instincts are strongest when the baby is at his most dependent.

Others feel that very new babies do little but eat, sleep, and cry, and think that for the first month or so babies need attention primarily for feeding, cleaning, and comforting. Some new parents feel that their very new babies are rather unrewarding companions: they seldom smile, their eyes wander, they don't reach out to people, they don't gurgle in recognition or even laugh when tickled. This is strictly true. However, what new babies can do is limited but can be endearing if you know where to look: any tiny baby will curl his hand around your finger if you touch his palm; many will visibly relax if you stroke their feet, or legs, or foreheads; some will push their feet against your hands if you do 'cycling' or 'knee-bending' exercises for them while they are lying down; they seem to fit almost miraculously into the crook of your arm of the curve of your tummy or the hollow of your neck and shoulder. If you put your hand on your baby's back or abdomen you can feel his stuttery, feathery breathing; if you put a (clean) finger into his mouth you can feel the power of his sucking reflex; if you watch him sleeping, or sometimes if you sing or talk while he is asleep you can see him making the same wriggling movements which he made before he was born.

Appreciating a tiny baby means understanding that he is in the first month or so making tremendous adjustments, and then watching for the responses he can make. His repertoire will expand, and will move from the instinctive responses of the first weeks to the intentional interaction of the later.

Restless babies   Some babies are more excitable than others and some lead an energetic and extrovert social life almost from the start. If you have this sort of baby it is sensible to adapt your life to his and be prepared to take him around with you, in a sling or on an adjustable seat, as you work. As babies get older they like to have something to watch, but bear in mind that interesting sights are no substitute for interesting company. You may like to keep the baby in the room with you all day, whatever you are doing. There is no reason for him to be banished to a far-away bedroom, like an invalid, when he sleeps.

Babies all over the world are carried on their mothers' bodies and the evidence seems to suggest that this keeps them snug and feeling secure. In the Western world, baby slings are becoming popular, both for ease of transport and to provide psychological comfort for restless babies. It is no reflection on you, however, if you have the sort of baby who loathes being handled and prefers a more solitary existence. If your baby cries constantly, you could try carrying him around in a sling during the day, as you do things around the house. This will not make him extra-dependent on you in later life, but will help give him a secure start, and he will soon feel confident enough to tackle independence. If your baby tends to bring up mouthfuls of stale-smelling milk when held upright in a sling, he (and your clothes!) might do better if you put him in a baby sling where he lies across your body instead. Encourage him to sleep between feeds. The NCT does not recommend carrying a baby under 12 weeks old in an upright sling for more than an hour or two at a time; and of course, at any age, you can carry your baby only until your own back or shoulders ache. There is, however, a new type of baby carrier available, where the baby is supported under his thighs as well as round his bottom, and this is safe to use from birth onwards.

Ailments

You will find many specialist books which discuss childhood ailments in detail. It is always difficult to gauge the seriousness of childhood ailments, especially with a first child and particularly in the middle of the night. You should not hesitate to contact your GP if you are really worried.

However, mothers with medical or paramedical backgrounds should guard against magnifying their children's ailments out of all proportion. When you are familiar with the symptoms of serious disease it is easy to imagine that your own baby's illnesses are more severe than they really are.

Practising

As prospective parents you may want to use visits to relatives and friends with babies or small children as discreet 'practice sessions', perhaps taking the children out for the afternoon or looking after the baby on your own for a time. Do find out about your local NCT gatherings so that you have a further opportunity of meeting mothers and babies and making friends. You will be welcome whether or not you have a baby in your arms. Valuable though these 'dummy runs' may be, do not allow yourselves to be overwhelmed or put off by the children's behaviour. Your own family will arrive one at a time (usually!) and you will be the ones to decide their lifestyle.

The ill and premature baby

Some babies are born needing special care. There are many reasons—some of the more common ones are described below —but most mean that the baby will go to a 'special care baby unit' to ensure that he receives the extra medical attention he requires.

Keeping in touch

When the baby is in a special care unit both parents should visit as much as possible. Do not be intimidated by all the equipment, and do not feel that you will be in the way, no matter how often you visit. The nursing and medical staff are there to help you and your baby. If he is ill in the incubator, reach in and hold his hand and comfort him. Talk to him so that he gets to know the sound of your voice. Once he is better you can take him out and give him a cuddle, and some units will let you give the tube feeds. Always ask the staff of the unit to explain what all the bits of apparatus do, since they will always appear somewhat strange and perhaps frightening to you when you first see them.

There is of course no reason why your special care baby should not benefit from your milk, in fact breast milk and colostrum are of particular value to him. From the start, learn to use a breast pump (see pp. 189 and 221) to express your milk which can then be given to your own baby. If there is any surplus it can be used to benefit other babies. Once your baby weighs about 1.7 kg (3¾ lb) and is well, he will be transferred to a cot, and when you come in you will be able to bathe and change him and establish him on breastfeeding. When the doctors judge that he is well enough, you will be able to take him home.

Small babies

Small-for-dates babies   These babies are mature but weigh less than normal for their length of gestation, and they can usually go with their mothers to the postnatal ward. However, because they are small they have poor nutritional reserves which can cause the glucose level in their blood to become very low during the first 48 hours. If prolonged this can damage the brain and cause subsequent handicap. To detect it, the small-for-dates baby needs heel prick blood tests for glucose estimations three to four times a day during the first 48 hours. During this period he can go to the breast to get the benefit of colostrum, but since you will be producing very little milk he will need to have complementary bottle feeds to prevent his blood glucose getting too low. Ask if he can have milk-bank breast milk rather than a formula. Occasionally (although rarely) this fails to keep the glucose level up and intravenous glucose will have to be given. Once lactation is established the baby can transfer to full breastfeeding.

Premature babies Babies of less than 2 kg (4½ lb) birthweight or less than 34 weeks' gestation usually need to be admitted to a special care baby unit. It is important to remember that although your baby is in the special unit, he is an entirely healthy little human being, and only needs to be there because of his environmental and feeding requirements.

In the unit, many babies are in incubators to keep them warm, to facilitate giving extra oxygen if necessary, and to make it easier for the nurses to keep a close watch on them in case their condition alters. Many premature babies, due to their immaturity, breathe irregularly and may even stop breathing, although they are otherwise completely well. They are therefore routinely laid on an 'apnoea' mattress (apnoea means 'no breathing') which sounds an alarm if the baby stops breathing, thus calling the nurse to come and stimulate him to breathe again before any harm is done.

Most babies under 34 weeks' gestation cannot suck on a nipple (yours or a bottle's) and need to be fed every two hours through fine plastic tubes passed through their noses into their stomachs, so that they do not have to make an effort to get food.

Sick premature babies With good management most of these babies now survive without any long-term handicaps. Between 28 and 30 weeks (when the baby weighs about 1 to 1.5 kg (2¼–3¼ lb) he has an 80 per cent chance of surviving, and more than 19 in 20 babies of more than 30 weeks' gestation and 1.5 kg (3¼ lb) birthweight will survive.

(a) Hyaline membrane disease, or respiratory distress syndrome (RDS) These are two names for one disease which is very common in premature babies. It develops within four hours of birth, and happens because the baby has immature lungs. Other than giving extra oxygen there is no specific treatment for the baby, who has to be helped to get over the illness himself, especially by giving him extra oxygen. The disease lasts five to

seven days, and once resolved leaves no after-effects. If it is known in time that the baby is to be born prematurely, then it is possible for the mother to receive injections which will help the baby's lungs to mature.

During the illness frequent checks on the level of oxygen and various other chemicals in the baby's blood will be made by passing a fine plastic tube (catheter) into his bloodstream through his umbilicus. This does not hurt or disturb the baby, and is used for taking blood and giving intravenous fluid or blood transfusions when necessary.

Around your baby's incubator will be various machines to record his heart-rate and respiration from electrodes fixed to his chest, to record the concentration of oxygen he is breathing, and infuse accurately small amounts of fluid through the umbilical catheter. The 10 per cent of these babies who have the worst lung disease will need a ventilator.

(b) Jaundice   Many babies develop jaundice at around three or four days old. This rarely does any harm, but very high levels can cause brain damage. If there is a risk of this, the baby needs to be put to the breast more frequently. If this does not control the jaundice he will be placed naked under bright lights to break down the yellow pigment in his skin (phototherapy). His eyes will be covered to protect them from the bright light. When you breastfeed him the eye covering can be removed.

(c) Other illnesses   Any illness, such as pneumonia or convulsions, can occur in a new baby, and will necessitate admission to the special care baby unit.

The malformed baby

One in about forty children is born with some malformation. Many of these are satisfactorily corrected by an operation but about 15 per cent of the malformed babies die shortly after birth, with some condition that cannot be treated.

If your baby has a malformation the medical staff will come and talk with both of you if possible soon after the delivery to explain the situation. You will be bewildered and miserable, and very little of what is said the first time will make sense, so do not be afraid to ask to see them again so that all your questions may be answered.

With some malformations the baby will be ill and admitted to the special care baby unit. You should always go and visit him, even if the condition is very likely to be fatal. If it is not, an operation may correct all his problems, and like any other newborn child he needs his mother and father from start. With many of these malformations you will be encouraged to look after your baby yourself, and he will be on the postnatal ward with you.

Babies requiring special care—how to cope—breastfeeding

Much of the information in this section applies to any situation when a mother wishes to maintain her breast-milk supply. In particular, it deals with pre-term babies. For babies in special care for other reasons, such as (2)–(7) below, additional advice on feeding needs and difficulties is best obtained from the staff who are caring for your baby, self-help groups for specific problems, and NCT breastfeeding counsellors.

Such situations could include:

1. pre-term birth,
2. hospitalization of your baby,
3. severe jaundice, requiring phototherapy,
4. physical handicap, for example cleft palate,
5. cot nursing, for example after a difficult birth or a forceps delivery,
6. small-for-dates babies,
7. ill babies and post-operative babies.

This section should be read in conjunction with pp. 179–81.

You and your baby

Many mothers find it comforting to provide breast milk for their baby if he is in a special care nursery as they feel it is the one thing only they can do, when everyone else has taken over the job of caring for him. Even if your baby is seriously ill, you will feel you are doing something worth while and positive for his care, if you express your milk. This is a very personal decision and you should be happy with whatever you decide to do. If you do not continue breastfeeding, for whatever reason, remember that even a small amount of breast milk will have benefited your baby.

Visit your baby often, touch him and talk to him as much as possible, so that you will get to know him and he will get to know you.

You may feel unhappy about being amongst mothers with their healthy babies in the postnatal ward—this is natural—but do talk about it and try to look forward to having your baby at home. Take the opportunity to get as much rest as possible. Use your relaxation techniques to calm your mind and relax your body.

Find out what times are best to visit your baby in the special care baby unit (SCBU) but make sure you don't miss your meals or medication on the postnatal ward. If your mealtime coincides with your baby's feed time, ask Sister to keep your food warm for you.

Do not be distressed when your baby is nursed in an incubator. Although it looks like a spaceship, it is little more than an open cot with plastic sides and top. This means that the nurses can observe your baby easily at all times—even from a distance—and slight changes in his colour or breathing pattern can be detected at once. If he was covered up with blankets in a cot, the nurses would have to disturb him frequently to monitor his condition. With your baby in an incubator you will probably be able to put your hands through the portholes to touch him and talk to him. Even if you can't do that, you will be able to watch him moving and will feel closer to him by being able to see him more clearly.

Often small and sick babies need the help of modern technology and there may be several machines connected to your baby. Most of these are monitors which enable the doctors and nurses to tell at a glance how your baby is doing. Do ask them to explain what each machine does; you may find it more fascinating than frightening. In time, as your baby does not need the machines, you will feel a sense of progress as he gradually manages on his own.

Communicating with hospital staff

Always share your feelings with your husband or partner; find out how he feels, and then together discuss your feelings and problems with the medical staff, who are there to help and inform you. If at first you don't understand your baby's treatment, ask more questions, or ask them to repeat their explanations. They know it is hard to take things in after the shock of a premature birth. Through the staff on the unit, make a special appointment with your baby's paediatrician for a full run-down on the treatment he is being given. It is very important for you to be fully informed and to understand everything in order to set your mind at rest. You will probably want to see the paediatrician more than once, and should be able to see him or her as often as you need to, within reason. Do not be afraid to ask questions or to admit that you don't understand something.

Family relationships and emotional support

If you are discharged before your baby, fitting in hospital visits, using the breast pump, making time for other children and your husband, not to mention getting adequate food and rest, will keep you very busy. Try not to let all this weigh you down. Take the opportunity to get out of the house, meet friends, and have an evening out with your husband or partner. Husbands can feel very left out when you are giving so much of your time and energy to feeding and visiting your baby.

Do try to have a 'quiet time' together each day so that you can develop the emotional support you need from each other. Many couples feel disorientated having a pre-term infant and often need to discuss their feelings with each other and also with friends or relatives. It is important to recognize these feelings and talk about them, before resentment builds up.

Many mothers feel very emotional after they have given birth, and with the added strain of being separated from your baby you are bound to feel depressed at times. A good cry can be a safety-valve to let out worry, frustration, and resentment. Remember, men can feel very emotional too and often they will need to cry to break the tension caused by the family situation. This is a normal emotional reaction, and better than having it all pent up, intensifying inside.

It may be difficult for you to accept a baby with whom you have had little physical contact. He may seem more like an object in a glass case than a cuddly little baby, especially if he is surrounded by wires and machinery. Don't be alarmed if you have few motherly feelings—these usually develop once you can hold and feel your baby and he becomes more responsive. It will probably take a little longer than usual, but when you have him at home with you he will feel more as though he belongs to you than to a hospital. Your feelings are normal. Be aware of them and talk about them. Don't bottle them up and worry about them. You may also have a 'delayed reaction' and feel the need to discuss your feelings some weeks after the birth.

Your other children may feel resentment towards this new baby to whom you are giving so much attention. Try to let them visit the hospital and see their new baby brother or sister. If you can arrange it with the Sister on the SCBU let them go into the unit to see and possibly touch their baby. It can be a good idea for a child to buy the baby a small present, such as a cuddly little toy which can be hung up near the incubator. This can be helpful in getting them to accept the new baby and you can gently explain to them why their baby brother or sister has to stay in hospital.

Looking after yourself

It is important for you to look after yourself and below are a few guide-lines to help you do this.

Avoid smoking and smoky atmospheres. Avoid alcohol. Do not take drugs or medication without your doctor's advice and whenever you consult him remind him that you are breastfeeding. It is best to use a method of contraception other than the pill whilst you are breastfeeding your baby.

Check that you eat regularly and that your diet is healthy and well balanced with adequate nourishment. A breastfeeding mother needs additional energy, about 500 K calories per day. See p. 243 for further discussion of diet. It is advisable to have something to drink and eat, such as a cup of tea and sandwich, each time you express your milk. This ensures you get extra food energy and fluid and helps you relax while expressing.

Breastfeeding

Breast milk is the best food for nearly all newborn babies. It is especially suited to your pre-term baby because he has an immature digestive system and, due to his small size and early arrival, he is particularly vulnerable to infection. Breast milk contains protective factors which help to protect your baby from infection and allergy. Recent research has shown that breast milk from mothers of pre-term babies is higher in protein than breast milk from mothers of full-term babies. This higher protein content helps your little baby's growth and development.

If your baby is very tiny (i.e. 1.5 kg (3¼ lb) or less), the paediatrician may prefer him to have a special formula feed. Other paediatricians will recommend supplements to breast milk to ensure that your baby is getting the best possible nutrition for his needs.

Establishing breastfeeding

On the delivery table you will probably be able to hold your baby for a short time. If he is very premature it will not be possible to suckle immediately after birth, so try not to feel too disappointed. He needs prompt medical attention because he may have some breathing difficulties and must be kept warm. Have a little cuddle and talk to him. Send a message to the Sister in charge of the SCBU that you plan to breastfeed your baby and, if possible, would like him given expressed breast milk (EBM) only.

Tell the Sister on your postnatal ward that you wish to breastfeed and she will help you to express your milk or show you how to use a hand breast pump or an electric one. You can start expressing very soon after the birth if your medical condition allows. Severe high blood pressure or having had a Caesarean section may delay starting but does not mean that you cannot feed at all. The first 'milk' you express is called colostrum. There is only a little of it but it is a very high-protein, concentrated food, which is the ideal transitional food for your baby. It also contains protective factors which will help to prevent infections and give him a good start.

Due to his prematurity and immature sucking and swallowing reflexes, it is unlikely that your baby will initially be able to feed directly from the breast. It will be necessary to express your milk and it will be given to him by tube. The tube goes through the baby's nose and into his stomach and is left in place between feeds. It is replaced by a clean one regularly. Sometimes the milk is given as a continuous feed with the help of a small electric pump. This method of feeding makes it possible for your baby to get his food without expending energy, so all the food goes into his growth.

Try to arrange to express your milk every three hours so that you are expressing *at least* four times a day—more often if possible. In this way your breasts will be stimulated to produce enough milk. Your milk should be given direct to your baby, without any treatment, by tube, until he is able to breastfeed. However, some hospitals prefer to treat the milk in some way before giving it to the baby. Ask for your milk to be kept especially for your own baby.

If you are not supplying sufficient milk for your baby's needs at first, it will be mixed with EBM from the hospital milk bank. If your hospital cannot provide EBM, it may be possible for the local branch of the NCT to do so. Small babies need relatively more food than full-term, average-weight ones, so don't be too depressed if you are not producing enough in the beginning.

See pp. 187–90 for details of the different ways of expressing milk.

Some hints on using electric breast pumps

Firstly, wash your hands and make sure all equipment has been sterilized. Always set the pump to the minimum suction setting. As the breasts get used to the sensation of using the machine, usually after a few minutes, gradually turn the suction up—you don't get much suction at minimum. Make sure you are adequately covered with protective towels to catch any spills. Always follow the instructions supplied with the pump. Always turn off the suction before removing the cup. Sore nipples can be a problem to anyone—see p. 182 for advice on how to cope.

It is important to relax as much as possible and many mothers find a photo of the baby helps them while expressing. If no photo is available, imagine that you are actually feeding your baby and try to 'think milk'. Sometimes a cassette tape of your favourite music helps, or even chewing gum. Some women watch TV or read a magazine. An occasional glass of sherry or other small alcoholic drink can help relaxation, but check with your baby's doctor if it would be wise. Your baby may be too weak or ill to tolerate even second-hand alcohol. A hot bath, or warm flannel applied to the breasts, or a little gentle massage will stimulate the 'let-down reflex'.

Find out how much your baby needs. You will be surprised what a small amount it is at first, but gradually he will want more and your breasts will produce what he needs, providing they receive enough stimulation from frequent expressing. In other words, 'little and often' is the catch-phrase to remember. Pumping three-hourly for five minutes each side, and use of the hospital pump whilst visiting, will produce more milk than fifteen minutes each side four-hourly. Try to express during the evenings and first thing in the morning as well. Find out your baby's feed times and pump at these times; it may make you feel closer.

Get into a routine of using the pump as soon as possible in the hospital. It is probably best to express when you wake, and then at three-hourly intervals until you go to bed. Five minutes each side at each of these sessions should be adequate. If you are only able to pump four times a day at roughly four-hourly intervals, try to hand express in between time for added stimulation. These are only suggested times, of course, and you must find a routine which suits your individual circumstances best.

When you are at home, set up the pump in a quiet, convenient place which gives you the amount of privacy you require. This will help you to use it with the minimum of fuss and bother. It is nice to have a helpful person around who will gather all your pump equipment together for you at each session, and wash up and sterilize it afterwards. Always remember that the pump is a means to an end, and that the end is 'normal' breastfeeding without the aid of a pump, or any bottles of any kind.

Adequate food and rest are also important. If you can get someone to take the pressure off you by doing some housework and shopping, don't refuse their help. Try to catnap in the day, and keep to simple nutritious meals. A breastfeeding mother needs additional energy, about 500 k calories. A glass of water or fruit juice or a cup of tea at every pump session, with a sandwich or snack, will keep up your fluid and energy intake and help you relax. Brewers' yeast tablets may also be helpful and are available from chemists. It is wise to check with your baby's doctor before taking any medicine which might affect your milk.

Gradual progression from pump to breast

Never compare breastfeeding a premature baby with breastfeeding a full-term baby. The management in the early days and weeks is quite different due to the baby's inability to suck well, his low weight, and his usually sleepy nature. However, remember that a full-term baby will feed very frequently, so you need to use the pump regularly.

When your baby is well enough to come out of the incubator for a short time you may be able to put him to the breast. The first time you hold your baby don't attempt to feed him, just have a cuddle and talk to him so you can get to know each other.

Try not to be nervous handling your baby. Physically he will be quite strong and emotionally he will be sensitive to your moods. He can sense if you are nervous, so try to be positive and look upon him as a little person with his own personality. Talk to him so he comes to recognize your voice.

At the first feed, don't expect too much, as the baby has to learn how to suck and will tire easily. If he has been having bottle-feeds, he has to relearn how to suck from the breast. Bottle-feeding and breastfeeding are different actions and different muscles will be used. You will notice the tops of the baby's ears wiggling when he is on the breast and sucking correctly. A few minutes will be enough the first time unless he gets the hang of it quickly and is obviously enjoying a good feed. Continue your pump routine even when the baby is breastfeeding, as his stimulation alone may not be sufficient to keep up your milk supply. Feed the baby first, when your breasts will be full, and after the feed express as usual. This expressed milk will be given to your baby by bottle or tube when you are not there.

When you are discharged you will probably be able to visit hospital for only one or two feeds daily, so do continue to express your milk at home and bring it to the hospital each day so that it can be given to your baby in your absence. Ask your midwife or health visitor to tell you how to collect and store your milk between visits and see 'How to express and store breast milk', p. 186.

Test weighing can be very trying and is almost inevitable in most SCBUs. For a period of twenty-four hours or so, your baby will be weighed before and after each breastfeed in an attempt to establish the amount of milk consumed at each feed. It is a way of trying to match baby's needs and feeds. When you are breastfeeding a little, giving some EBM by bottle, and the remainder is given by tube to your very sleepy baby, it often seems to be too much bother. Try to regard this difficult period as a passing phase and continue to be single-minded, determined, and dedicated; take one day at a time and try not to become impatient over slow progress.

When it is near the long-awaited day of your baby's home-coming, try to arrange a full day at the hospital when you can breastfeed for every feed without 'topping-up'. Some hospitals have a system where mothers can come in two/four days before their baby goes home. Ask what the system is in your hospital. Ask if it would be possible for your baby to wear his own clothes in hospital before he comes home. Some hospitals encourage this practice. Do remember to continue using the pump, or to hand express after feeds. Ask the hospital to keep any surplus milk frozen, or store it in your own freezer, in case you need it once you get home. If you don't, you can always donate it for use in the SCBU. Remember your baby may not be as 'old' as a full-term baby even now, and will need shorter, more frequent feeding for a time as his stomach capacity is small. Most premature babies are prescribed iron medicine, as they are born before they had time to lay down iron reserves in their livers.

Encouraging a reluctant baby to suck

There are several little 'tricks' you can use to help your baby suck:

1. Hand expressing a little milk can help the nipple to stand out and make it easier for the baby to fix.

2. Expressing is also helpful if your breasts are full or you have a slow 'let-down reflex'.

3. Warm compresses can help the let-down reflex.

4. If you are very anxious, your let-down can be encouraged by using syntocinon nasal spray. This is available on prescription and can tide you over difficult times.

5. Some mothers find a latex nipple shield helpful (available from the NCT), and if you have flat nipples it can be useful as it offers the baby something to latch on to at first.

6. Babies will sometimes take more interest if the nipple has a little breast milk or glycerine applied before a feed.

7. A teat with a 'natural' shape can be used with bottles of EBM, or there are alternative shapes which your baby may find easier to grasp.

8. If your baby has a problem latching on, there is an aid consisting of a small plastic bag intended to contain your expressed breast milk plus a long flexible plastic tube which you tape to your nipple. The baby thus gets his feed of EBM and learns to suck from the breast and stimulates your supply at the same time. This can be helpful when getting the baby on to the breast, but do not use it unless it is necessary: the less paraphernalia you have to cope with the better.

At home When you have your baby home with you don't stop using the pump, unless you have already established satisfactory demand feeding. Continue using the pump to give adequate stimulation to your breasts in order that they produce sufficient milk. Use the excess milk to 'top up' this way for a week or two, or maybe a little longer, until your baby is used to sucking efficiently at the breast for all his nourishment.

Try not to become so dependent on the pump that you feel you cannot breastfeed without it. It is an aid for you to use as you need it and the sooner you can do without it the easier feeding will become.

If you decide to stop breastfeeding, or have to stop for a medical reason, there is no need to feel guilty or a failure. Your baby can be given a suitable alternative. You will find it more comfortable to express once or twice a day until your supply dwindles. This EBM can be used to feed other babies in the SCBU—unless you are on drugs or have an infection. Cold compresses help to cut down the milk supply. Very occasionally your doctor will prescribe tablets to dry up your milk.

During the day, when it is easier to give short, frequent feeds, try dropping the top-up, one feed at a time. Only top up at night when you want feeds to be shorter and quickly satisfying so that you don't miss too much sleep. Use your own judgement. You may find he does not need top-ups after a few days.

Take every opportunity to relax and sleep, and accept any offers of help. Also try short feeds even when your baby is not very hungry as this sucking practice will be good for him and stimulate milk production in the breasts.

It takes time to establish breastfeeding in a full-term baby, so be patient and dedicated when attempting to feed your pre-term baby. Lean heavily on your husband, family, and friends for support, and you will feel a great sense of achievement when you are at last 'normally' breastfeeding your baby.

Stillbirth

Whether a baby is stillborn or dies just after birth you will be numbed by what has happened. Why me? Why us? You will want to know the answers to many questions: Was it something we did? Will it happen again? Your obstetrician, paediatrician, and general practitioner will often be able to answer these questions for you and you may need to see them several times before you get a full grasp of what has happened. Remember that the paediatrician usually wants to do a post-mortem on the baby. This may not only help him to prevent another baby dying of the same condition, but without it he may not be able to answer the question 'Will it happen again?'

If you know in advance that your baby will be stillborn, the staff will do their best to help you through the experience. You will probably discuss with them beforehand whether or not you and your partner will want to hold the baby when he is born. With this, as with other choices you will be given, you will be asked again later and can, of course, change your minds if you wish.

During the labour you and your partner will share unique parental grief and will start the process of mourning. Spare a thought for the midwife who will be sharing your feelings to a great extent, but who has to control her emotions in order to conduct the labour skilfully.

Whether or not the stillbirth is anticipated, you will probably be reassured by the baby's normal appearance if you do decide to hold him. Holding the baby can help you come to terms with his death and to understand his reality as a person. When you remember and grieve for him, he will not be an unseen 'fantasy baby'. You may prefer to be left alone together with the baby for a short time. One father of a stillborn baby sketched a picture of her, and the whole family drew comfort from the acknowledgement of her life. A photograph might be an alternative to a drawing. Some hospitals routinely take a photograph and you can have a copy at a later date, should you wish.

You may wish to recognize the baby's individuality by giving him a name. Unpleasant though it is, you will have to register the birth and the death of your child. There may be a registrar of births and deaths at the maternity hospital and the nursing staff will help you with the arrangements. You will need to discuss funeral arrangements and the hospital staff will again be able to help you contact a local funeral director, if you want a private funeral. Otherwise, the hospital will be able to arrange a burial.

A breastfeeding counsellor can advise on ways of alleviating any discomfort in your breasts. You may even like to express your colostrum to help save the life of another dangerously ill baby.

Attitudes to stillbirth

Some people think that after a stillbirth the parents should forget all about it and think about other things. This rarely succeeds in erasing painful memories and can interrupt the process of grieving. Mourning is the natural, normal response to loss and there are no short cuts to bypass the experience.

In hospital you may prefer to be in a single room, away from other mothers and their newborn babies. If there is no single room available, you may be put in a ward containing a number of other mothers who are separated from their babies for one reason or another, so that you do not have to bear this deprivation alone.

Some bereaved mothers feel that the hospital staff are not interested in them. This is very far from the truth. Often the staff desperately want to help but do not know what to do. They may feel that they are intruding or interfering in a private grief if they spend too much time with you; they may feel they have failed you by delivering a stillborn baby, even if the stillbirth was inevitable. Share your grief with them and, if you wish, particularly with the midwife who attended you in labour. She, too, will be mourning and will be under the strain of presenting a normal face to the other patients.

Try to use the stressful days after a stillbirth to express your grief and to begin the slow process of healing. Be considerate, in your distress, of those friends and relatives who sympathize deeply but do not know how to respond or to help you. If, in later conversation, people laboriously steer clear of the subject of your baby's death, their usual motive will be that of not wishing to bring back your painful memories and of not appearing to be inquisitive. They are not avoiding the subject because they do not care.

You may find it helpful to talk to someone who has experienced a stillbirth, and who can offer first-hand understanding and guidance. The Stillbirth and Neonatal Death Society can be contacted at Argyle House, 29–31 Euston Road, London NW1 2SD.

Some hints about twins

A few general ideas

The mother who has learned how to relax completely and how to use only those muscles necessary for each task is at a tremendous advantage in coping with twins. If you can get one hundred per cent value out of each minute of rest and avoid becoming flustered and panicky as jobs pile up, you will have fresh energy to cope even though you are bound to get very tired at times. Correct posture and working habits learned during pregnancy will enable you to avoid backache and the general weariness that comes from poor posture. It is most important that you remember to do your postnatal exercises.

Plan ahead to get a lying-down rest each day, and get a couple of really early nights each week even though it means waking to feed the babies. Try to adopt a relaxed attitude to the problems you encounter. All new babies really need is plenty of milk whenever they want it, cleanish clothes, an occasional wash, and lots of loving. With twins it is easy to aim at standards which are too high for everyone's comfort.

A helpful person—relative or friend—who can spend part of a day with you makes a great difference in the first month.

It is wise, not extravagant, to spend money on help in the house, and on disposable nappies or a nappy service, or a fully automatic washing machine. A tumble drier is perhaps the most useful of all. There is no need to buy any elaborate baby equipment. Second-hand twin prams are cheap, but you will need another cheap pram or carrycot on wheels after the first six weeks or so, since the babies will keep each other awake. A folding twin pram/push-chair with separate back-rests is very handy for shopping and outings. If you have to take the twins on a weekly shopping expedition, it may be helpful to choose a shopping area which is pedestrianized or has wide pavements, or to go to a large 'superstore' (preferably with a crêche where the babies can be supervised) where everything is under one roof.

Handle the babies as much as possible; you can never cuddle two babies as much as you could cuddle one. If you wish, take the babies to bed with you for an afternoon rest, making little nests for them in your bed, well free of blankets and pillows.

If you watch and closely observe your babies you will find that even identical twins are very different. It is this personal individuality which it is important to respect, loving each child for himself alone, not even for what he is in the family (the youngest or the eldest or one of the twins) or for what he might be if he were good all the time, but for himself, just as he is.

If possible have more clothing than you think you will need for the twins, even if they are cast-offs, so that when things really pile up you do not have to bother about washing and drying. It helps if the babies'—and the family's—clothes are made of drip-dry fabrics.

As they grow older many twins develop means of communication with each other which by-pass words, or even a special language which only the two of them understand. One child can be very distressed if a parent smacks the other, and on the whole this is best avoided.

Try not to leave the twins alone too often to amuse one another. Like all babies and children, they need the stimulus of frequent contact with an adult to help them develop skills in speech and social development.

You are bound to need means of keeping the babies within a confined range. There are several forms of baby bouncer on the market and one or two of these, or baby swings, hung out of harm's way in the kitchen will be useful for short periods after about four to six months. A playpen is almost essential. Once they are mobile, a light webbing harness on each baby can be quickly clipped in place on the high chair. In the garden you may wish to fence off a safe area using plastic-coated railing or plastic-coated strong wire netting.

You probably run more risk of accidents with two babies than with one, simply because you are busy and rushed. So plan ahead so that they cannot possibly topple out of highchairs or roll off beds.

Breastfeeding twins

Start breastfeeding as soon after birth as possible. Feed on demand if possible, at least three-hourly at first, letting each baby regulate his own intake. Frequent feeding of both babies stimulates the breast enough to supply milk for both babies. If you feed only one baby the stimulation is less and the breasts supply only enough milk for one baby.

Don't worry about timings: remember each baby is an individual and one may take longer to feed than the other. Many mothers have found it better to keep one breast for one baby rather than swop round at each feed. Each baby builds up his own supply on his own breast so that individual fluctuations of appetite can be catered for. You may feel a little 'lop-sided' at times if they vary much in demand, but it seems to settle down evenly after a couple of weeks.

You may find it easier to feed the babies separately at first so that you get to know each one as an individual and learn how to handle them and how to relax and enjoy feeding them. You may want to continue feeding your twins separately or you may find it easier to feed them together once you get the hang of it.

There are real advantages in feeding simultaneously. It takes less time when older children are around, less time at night, and is an advantage if both babies wake up hungry at the same

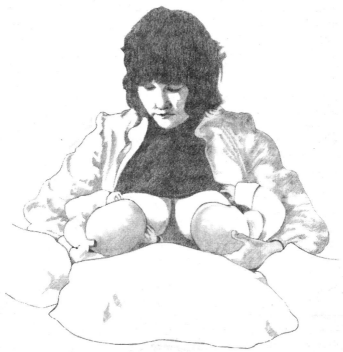

Breastfeeding twins simultaneously

time. A settee is the most comfortable place to feed your babies like this. You will need three pillows or cushions and something to wipe up dribbles. Place one pillow, to support their backs, on either side of where you intend to sit. Lay one baby safely on the settee and, holding the other baby in your arms, sit down, placing the third pillow on your lap. Lay one baby on each side, on his back, with the two heads close together on the pillow on your lap, so that their heads are just below your breasts. You may then hold the babies to the breast with your cupped hands under their heads, or adjust the pillow on your lap to support their heads. This leaves your hands free to wind each baby by turning him on to his tummy on the pillow where he may wind himself, or by raising him gently while the other continues feeding.

There may be times when you need to build up your milk supply, so breastfeed every two or three hours for a day or so. Remember to eat and drink plenty yourself. (Your calorie output will be increased by at least 1,500 calories in the form of milk production.)

Bottle-feeding twins

Make sure that both babies get sufficient cuddling and enough of your handling and attention. Don't be tempted to hand one twin for feeding to anyone who happens to be around. As far as possible make feeding your job and use all the help you can for other chores. Simultaneous feeding means simultaneous hunger. It is much easier to get the babies going roughly one behind the other so there is time to get to know each one separately, and to have a hand free for a toddler.

If the twins are very tiny and need 2–3 hourly feeds you may find that you have to feed them together or you will literally never stop feeding. If you are feeding alone at night you will probably find that you will never get any sleep if you demand-feed entirely. Wake the second baby after finishing the first. If your husband is willing to get up at night to help with feeding you might find doing alternate nights each is better than both being up at every feed, or you could do alternate feeds each.

It is possible to bottle-feed two babies together by yourself, although it is not easy. Sit on a bed or settee and prop one baby in the corner supported by cushions, holding his bottle in your left hand; cuddle the second baby with his head in the crook of your right arm, your right arm reaching in front of him to hold his bottle. This ensures that one baby gets some cuddling and you can alternate the one you hold at each feed.

Try not to get into the habit of propping both babies on cushions and just holding the bottles. This means that the babies miss out on close contact with you, and the temptation to prop up the bottles as well and get on with seemingly urgent tasks is great. This is a really dangerous thing to do because the babies can easily choke.

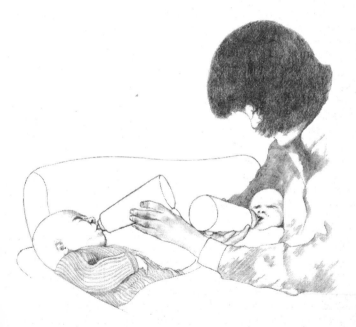

Bottle-feeding twins simultaneously

Make up feeds for 24 hours at a time and refrigerate them; it saves time and there is much less chance of contamination. A plastic bucket or bread bin makes a good sterilizing unit for the number of bottles you will be using.

Solid foods

When you introduce solid foods it is easiest to place the babies' high chairs close together (but not so close that they smother each other with food) and feed them alternately out of one bowl, either with the same spoon or with a spoon in each hand. Twins soon learn to feed each other, and each may find it simpler to put food in the other's mouth rather than his own!

Some mothers of twins, in an understandable attempt to save time, make the mistake of feeding their children exclusively on manufactured baby foods long after they could cope with ordinary meals. You will save money, and help the twins' adjustment to eating solid foods, if you give them small portions of the family's meals, puréed, mashed, or chopped as appropriate. There may be a Twins Club in your area where you could meet other families and share ideas.

Adopted babies

Adoption is a large subject which can only be touched on briefly, so mention is made here of only a few points which adoptive parents have found to be of particular importance or to be less well covered in the existing literature. There are a number of books available from public libraries outlining legal procedures and discussing in full various practical and emotional factors which couples considering adoption would do well to think over before they approach an adoption agency. Once in contact with an agency (or with your local authority) you will, of course, have the help and support of the social worker handling your case and of the health visitor when a baby finally arrives.

The first few days

It is difficult to generalize about adopted babies because they are individuals who respond to life in their own very personal ways. Frequently, however, they do have a rather different start to life from the majority, arriving at the home of their adoptive parents after a period in hospital and often after some weeks or even months with foster parents. A baby is very sensitive to his environment from birth onwards and may well show some distress for a few days after his arrival at his adoptive parents' home. He will have come to depend for comfort and reassurance on his foster mother and will be accustomed to the sights and sounds of daily life in her home, so do not be surprised if the baby, who—you had been assured —was a model of good behaviour, is at first restless and distressed. Natural parents often have a similar experience on returning home with their new babies! This will be an anxious time for you if this is your first baby so, like other mothers, you will need to give as much time as you can spare to relaxing and enjoying the baby and put your own need to rest before the demands of housekeeping. If after a few days your baby still seems unduly troubled, your health visitor will be glad to give you guidance and reassurance, and you may well find that sharing your own maternal experience with friends and rela-tives or with the members of the NCT postnatal support group is a great aid in bolstering your morale.

From your point of view the arrival of your long-awaited baby may come as a bit of a shock. You may be taking this small stranger into your family after the briefest of introductions and without nine months' biological preparation which to the natural mother often seems over-long. Even if you are sure, within yourself, that you have great wells of maternal love just waiting to be released, your emotions in the hours following the baby's arrival may savour more of panic and a feeling that the world has turned a somersault, than of glowing motherly pride. Some adoptive parents feel that a little previous contact with their baby—a couple of visits to the foster home, for instance

—helped them to ease themselves more gently into their new role, and gave the wife the chance to begin to see herself as the baby's mother. A husband, too, may be unsure that he will be able to love someone else's child as well as his own, so he might also appreciate the opportunity to get to know the baby step by step. It might, therefore, be sensible to ask your social worker if one or two preliminary visits to the foster parents could be arranged.

You will soon come to know your baby intimately and as you do your love for each other will grow; indeed many mothers only 'fall in love' with their babies gradually over the early weeks, so do not feel ashamed if it turns out to be a gradual process for you.

Breastfeeding an adopted baby

Sometimes an adoptive mother longs to experience the close, loving relationship which can come from nursing a baby at the breast. It may come as a surprise to her to hear that this is not physiologically impossible, even for a woman who has never been pregnant. The stimulation of the breast by suckling can be sufficient to trigger off the secretion in the mother's body of the hormone prolactin, responsible for the production of breast milk. Trying to breastfeed an adopted baby is very hard work, but it can be very rewarding. A woman who has not recently given birth will probably not be able to fulfil all her baby's nutritional needs because her breasts have not been stimulated by pregnancy; nonetheless it is often possible to build up a milk supply after persuading the baby to suckle at an initially dry breast. And there lies the catch: although some babies will suck anything with gusto, most find it unrewarding to suckle at an unproductive breast (for a period varying from a few days to several weeks) before even a trickle of milk appears. There is a gadget which consists, very simply, of a bag for the milk formula, or expressed breast milk (EBM), which is suspended round the mother's neck on a cord, to which is attached a length of very fine tube which lies against the breast to end at the mother's nipple. The baby can then receive his milk supply while suckling at the breast, giving him a reward for his efforts which will make him work harder. It is not so simple and straightforward to use as a baby's bottle, and is an awkward shape for cleaning, so it might not be worth the extra trouble for a baby who will suckle at breast or bottle without preference. Unlike a normal lactation, breastfeeding an adopted baby will involve a mother in more rather than less work: a factor which might deter someone who has other children in the family or who feels that it is going to take her all her time to care for her baby anyway. If, however, you feel that the mutual pleasure of nursing and the benefit to the baby that even a small amount of breast milk would bring would repay your initial effort, you are advised to contact the NCT some time before a baby is offered to you, to seek further advice, and to arrange for a counsellor to be in touch to give you help and support after the baby's arrival. You may also like to discuss the matter with your social worker, who might be able to arrange for you to have a very young baby, since one who has become accustomed to a bottle over a number of weeks will be much less likely to take to the breast than a relatively new baby.

The older baby

It you are adopting an older baby, or a toddler, breastfeeding will not be a consideration, but developing a loving bond between you will be equally important. The newcomer may be wary of you at first and may seem to reject you at precisely those times when you most want to give him your comfort and love. If you are patient and respect his feelings, he will soon come to trust you; though having gained you, he will be particularly anxious not to let you slip. He may panic in your absence and be, for a while, unusually timid about venturing far from your side. It is tempting for parents to feel that these and other difficulties are peculiar to their child because he is adopted, but many natural parents have in special circumstances had similar experiences with their children. Once again, do not hesitate to discuss your problems with other people.

Existing children's reactions

The busiest adoptive mother will be the one whose baby joins an existing family of children. Your previous experience will, of course, stand you in good stead, but you must reckon that your other child or children—far from being extra helpful—may well be a little extra demanding of your time and patience for a while, in particular the one who was the 'baby' of the family before. If they are old enough, they will be aware to some extent of the adoption procedure and will be excited and proud to tell their friends about 'our adopted baby'. You must be careful not to give them to understand that the arrangement is permanent until the adoption is finalized, otherwise they will be greatly distressed if the baby has to be returned to his natural mother and it may make them wonder if their own place in the family is secure. It would be as well to decide, right from the start, how much you intend to let your children (or anyone else) know about your baby's previous history, bearing in mind that what you tell your children will soon be known to all the world! They will be satisfied with a few quite simple facts and there is no need to give them detailed information which would be better written down and put away for safe keeping until your adopted child is older. Don't delay in committing details of an adopted baby's background to paper; even months afterwards you will find it impossible to sort out in your mind between what your social worker actually told you and what you deduced from information you were given.

Consideration towards adoptive parents

Lastly, a word for those of you reading this section who are not and do not expect to be adoptive parents. Please be especially considerate of anyone you encounter who is in the process of adopting a baby. The procedure itself is long and arduous, and is by no means over when the baby comes home, as it may be many months before the adoption is finalized and the parents can at last relax and get rid of the feeling of being eternally 'on approval'. Sometimes they may have had to face criticism from their wider family (it is natural enough, for instance, for grand-parents to be anxious for the welfare of their other grand-children when a baby or especially a toddler is brought into an existing family), and they will be particularly appreciative if you give the newcomer a warm welcome and show yourself ready to share in their joy and pleasure. Finally, a childless couple will have experienced much sorrow and stress because of their infertility, which will not be dispelled immediately by the new arrival, however delightful he may be. His mother will still feel to some extent that she missed the experience of pregnancy and giving birth and will long to know about the baby's birth and what took place before his arrival in her home. While she needs and will welcome the company of other new mothers, she might not wish to be regaled with the saga of your 'birth experience'.

THE NEW
PARENTS

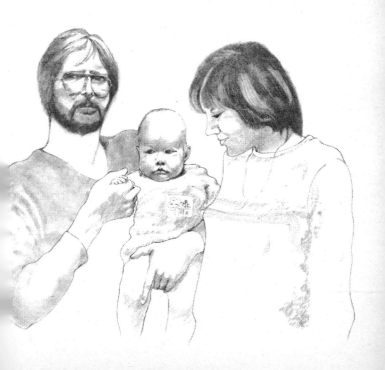

Introduction

The time immediately after the birth of a first baby is tradition-ally one for rejoicing, when grandparents and friends rally round and the new family becomes the centre of attention. Sometimes, however, the parents feel too stressed and unsure of themselves to enjoy these early days when everyone else seems so blissfully delighted. The relationship in the first six weeks or so between a mother and her new baby is very like the early days of a courtship or a honeymoon. Little drawbacks become magnified out of all proportion, while the pleasures are heightened into elation. It is a time of emotional extremes when your moods may swing from wonder and joy to helplessness and despair—all over things which, rationally, should cause you little concern. Be prepared for this, and enjoy the emotional 'highs' in all their intensity.

Here are a few practical points worth bearing in mind:

1. As a new mother, you need to eat sensibly to keep well and active, and to maintain your milk supply if you are breastfeeding.

2. Just as pregnancy may call for adjustments in your sexual life, so the period of change after the baby is born can also affect your lovemaking—particularly if you have had an episiotomy and are apprehensive about intercourse being painful.

3. While most women adapt very well to motherhood, a small number, through no fault of their own, suffer from postnatal depression in varying degrees of severity. Medical help should always be sought for this condition. It can be treated and should never be a cause for shame or embarrassment.

4. Caring for a small baby can be an isolating experience, particularly if you live a long way from other members of your family or know few people in your neighbourhood. NCT groups throughout the country run informal systems for post-natal support, for women who seek this type of self-help and companionship. There may be similar schemes run by other organizations, for example MAMA (Meet-a-Mum Association), or your health visitor.

5. It is important that the needs of each member of the new family are satisfied and respected. Mother, father, and children all have interdependent demands and you should work consciously to balance them, so that one person's desires do not become dominant.

Diet after the baby arrives

A good diet is important to keep a new mother healthy and thus able to look after her baby. Every new mother needs to eat well to have enough energy. If you are breastfeeding, you need to eat more to produce milk; even if you are bottle-feeding you need regular balanced meals or you will become over-tired and perhaps depressed. Eating something every two-and-a-half to three hours will help to raise the blood sugar level and keep depression at bay. For details of sources of essential nutrients, see p. 47.

Diet during breastfeeding

The breastfeeding mother is, indeed, eating for two. You will need more food than when you were pregnant. A baby consumes, on average, 600 calories a day.

Human milk is composed of protein, fat, carbohydrate (a special sugar called lactose), minerals, and vitamins. The protein can be provided by eating an extra 45 g (1½ oz) of meat or cheese or an extra half-pint of milk. The other nutrients in human milk can be made from carbohydrates: bread, potatoes, cereals, etc. Minerals and vitamins pass directly to the baby, so the mother's diet must contain enough for both of them.

If you are breastfeeding, your body will make milk for your baby before taking out your own nourishment, so protect your own health as well as your baby's by eating a well-balanced diet. Your milk supply is maintained by eating enough calories and by eating frequently. Do not miss meals, for you are making milk all the time. If your milk supply decreases, eat an extra snack or two: toast, a sandwich, or crispbread and cheese plus a drink at each feed is a good way to plan the extra food needed. The supply may adjust itself within a few hours. If you feel tired or depressed, eat small amounts more often (about every 2–3 hours) to keep up your blood sugar level. If you feel ill and go off your food, with a resultant reduction of milk, don't worry: it will increase again as soon as you resume your normal diet. In the mean time, have plenty of nourishing drinks or soups.

Forbidden foods?

Is there any food a breastfeeding mother cannot eat? Generally speaking, no—you can eat what you fancy. Some drugs pass unchanged into the milk, so consult your doctor about medicines. Babies do not usually react adversely to any food that their mothers eat while producing breast milk. Eat whatever you were eating during pregnancy, and avoid an excessive intake of new foods—a sudden spicy meal or too much fruit or chocolate. If you do not normally eat a particular food, try a small amount of a moderately seasoned portion first. Seasonal fruits may need 'breaking in' in this way. Do not avoid fruit, however. Both you and the baby need the vitamin C, and it helps to prevent constipation. Sometimes certain foods in the mother's diet do obviously affect the baby and you will need to avoid these.

Breastfeeding mothers get thirsty. You will need to drink more fluids than usual, and especially while feeding the baby. Any fluid will do; just follow your thirst and taste. Milk and stout are often recommended, but there is nothing magical about them. Milk does not make milk; it is simply a very good source of calories, protein, calcium, and other nutrients. Too much coffee or tea, incidentally, may reduce your milk supply, so drink these in moderation while establishing breastfeeding. Do not force yourself to drink, especially if you are worried that you haven't enough milk. There is some evidence to show that when mothers are forced to drink more water than they want, they produce less milk. If dairy products in your diet make your baby colicky or give him a rash, you will need to avoid cows' milk and cheese, but you may find that goats' milk is all right for you to use. A milk-free diet sheet is available from the NCT on receipt of a stamped addressed envelope.

Losing weight

You will probably be 3–6 kg (7–14 lb) over your pre-pregnancy weight after the baby is born. This is nature's way of providing a reserve to make milk. Do not try to diet while establishing breastfeeding—you are more likely to reduce the milk supply and exhaust yourself. The extra few pounds generally disappear during the first few months of looking after a new baby—and breastfeeding helps this process—or else after weaning the baby (as the hormones involved in breastfeeding cause water retention). Be sure to do postnatal exercises so that your muscles will be back into shape in preparation for your weight loss later. Sometimes pregnancy alters the body's metabolism and you may need to go on a slimming diet after weaning. Eating well, but not to excess, should be your rule while your baby is still new and you need all the energy you can get. Obviously avoid 'junk' food, refined or ready prepared foods, or those full of sugar, white flour, etc., but do eat plenty of wholegrain carbohydrates as recommended in the chapter on diet in pregnancy.

Sex after the baby is born

After the drama of labour it is wonderful to hold your newborn child in your arms and to realize that you are suddenly parents, even though it hardly seems believable. The sense of having as a couple shared the making of the baby can be very strong, and many couples find that the feeling of sharing continues throughout parenthood. Others, however, find that the baby becomes the focus of so much attention that its parents have trouble relating to each other except as parents, or that they spend so much time paying attention to the baby that they make too little time for themselves. It is rather like having a house-guest: when even a weekend visitor comes, for instance, couples can quickly find that they seldom see each other alone or when not preoccupied with the guest's needs or with the alterations the visit makes to their usual pattern of life. And, depending on the guest, you can find it easy or difficult to adjust. With congenial friends staying overnight after a special meal and relaxing evening, you may feel perfectly happy to leave dirty dishes for the morning and to retire to bed and make love just as you always do. Whereas with your parents-in-law you might not feel quite so uninhibited, either about leaving the dishes or about making love ('Not tonight, in case the bed creaks and disturbs them'). You become the model host and hostess, not your usual selves. In the same way, many couples react to the birth of their first baby by beginning to see themselves as the baby's mother and father more often than as a loving couple. But labour does not mysteriously turn a woman into a Mother Earth figure with no sexual desires, and fatherhood does not transform her partner into a man with only paternal feelings.

Many adjustments have to be made after the birth of a baby, and family relationships all shift in subtle ways as a new generation of parents—and grandparents—is created. The arrival of second and subsequent babies also causes changes.

The birth of a baby can place stress on even a happy partnership if the woman believes she is an undesirable drudge or the man feels neglected in favour of the baby. They may both feel they can never recapture the romance of courtship and the spontaneity of lovemaking.

Traditional attitudes

As with sex in pregnancy, traditions of many kinds linger on over the behaviour of new parents. In some cultures the woman receives special protection: she may be fed special foods and treated in a ritual manner. In other cultures, the father is thought to need special attention: in the custom known as the 'couvade', for instance, *he* goes to bed and is cossetted during or after his partner's labour. In this country, some women feel that they cannot take up their normal lives until after they have been 'churched'.

In many societies one of these traditions is a ban on inter-course for a specified period after childbirth. The reasons given vary, including fear of injuring the vagina or introducing infection to the uterus, and bear little relation to evidence of when any one woman feels physically capable of intercourse, which may be as soon as a week after a normal delivery. The length of advised abstinence differs from country to country: for instance, six weeks in the USA and three in France. In Britain opinions vary: some doctors say you should wait until after the six-week check, while others say you should be sure to recommence before the six-week check so that you can raise any problems at it.

Nevertheless, although a woman may be physically ready for sex very shortly after the birth of her child, she often feels in need of a period of sexual respite. However deeply she loves her partner, she may dislike the thought of making love or may lose interest once lovemaking has started. Almost without exception she will want her partner to give her extra care and attention. This may be a time when other expressions of love are appropriate.

Many men feel that for a time after the birth sex is inappropri-ate; it may just not feel 'right'. The birth may have been a profoundly moving experience, leaving them satisfied and enthralled or perhaps uneasy and disturbed. Just as the woman may feel like a 'vessel' which everyone else seems to have a use for, and need time to feel that her body is her own again, the man may need time to adjust to his partner as a mother.

Too tired

The old excuse 'I'm too tired' may be only too true for the new parents. The mother's day is filled with new experiences and new responsibilities so that in bed she longs only for the oblivion of sleep. She may be so tense and preoccupied that she is unable to get into the mood of mutual giving and receiving necessary for happy lovemaking. (Relaxation techniques can again be helpful.) The baby may be waking at night and refusing to settle. If either partner has been unable to sleep during the day because of work or the washing and cooking taking unwarranted precedence over rest, then he or she may not be as sympathetic and helpful as he or she might wish. It is easy to forget that sex at night is closely linked with behaviour during the day.

Sensitive spots

Making love after childbirth can be pretty uncomfortable. The natural vaginal lubrication may be absent at this time and the vagina itself may feel taut and dry. You may both find it helpful if the woman uses a lubricating jelly or cream (for instance a contraceptive cream or one sold for keeping the nipples supple) in her vagina and smooths some on her partner's penis before penetration.

If the woman has had stitches she will not only be sore, she will (unless she is a paragon of self-control) have negative memories of the episiotomy and suturing process and may subconsciously recoil from having such a sensitive place touched again. In the days immediately following the episiotomy the stitches may only 'prickle', or they may be so painful that practically every bodily movement pulls them. After this has passed, there is often a tender lump along the line of the incision for the next few months. Any pressure against this will be unpleasant and may be emphasized if the woman tenses and draws back in apprehension when her partner tries to enter her.

When making love after there has been a tear or an episiotomy it is important not only to make sure that there is enough lubrication but also to choose a position in which the penis presses on the clitoris and front wall of the vagina rather than against the tender area at the back. The woman will find it helpful to guide the man inside her while she deliberately releases her pelvic floor muscles. If intercourse continues to be painful in spite of consideration and gentle lovemaking, she should consult her obstetrician.

After birth the woman may find clitoral stimulation particularly enjoyable and should help her partner to discover exactly what gives her the most pleasure. You may both find that positions which before giving birth were perfectly acceptable are now associated by the woman with obstetric procedures and are consequently quite off-putting to her. Experimentation may be necessary until the memories fade.

If the woman is breastfeeding, her partner should be careful not to put pressure on her sensitive breasts. She will be especially milky and uncomfortable at night if the baby unexpectedly sleeps longer than usual between feeds. Sometimes when the breasts become sexually aroused they leak milk. To minimize this it is best to make love soon after a feed. Once again, you may need to try different positions for sex.

One, or both, of you may be inhibited about making love if the baby is in the same room. Put the child behind a screen or move him to another room.

Contraception

You may worry about starting another baby very soon, since contraceptives are not usually prescribed until the postnatal examination at six weeks. Breastfeeding usually inhibits ovulation but not always, so it is very unwise to rely on it as a form of contraception. The woman may not want to take the pill if she is breastfeeding, but if she does she should make sure it is the 'mini-pill' (progestogen only), which should not affect the hormones of lactation. However, it does go through the milk to the baby. The woman may find it makes her depressed. Some women find that if they take it before the milk supply is properly established, they just cannot increase their supply, even if they have breastfed previously. Her milk supply will probably be reduced for a couple of days after commencing it, but can usually pick up again if she feeds more frequently for 48 hours.

The man may use a sheath, but this may cause discomfort to a dry and tender vagina and will need to be used with a lubricating cream or jelly. If the woman used a cap before the baby was conceived she will find that it will now be too small, but smeared liberally with spermicide it should provide adequate protection until she can obtain another. If she has no cap, the best answer may be to insert a lot of spermicide into the vagina, near the cervix, with the applicator provided.

There are now centres where parents can learn about 'natural' family planning methods, and properly taught by a qualified teacher, these can be very successful.

Postnatal exercises

1. Several times daily, if you are confined to bed, and also each morning when you wake up and after your daily rest, circle your feet and then stretch and draw up your toes, in order to stimulate your circulation and tone up the muscles of your feet and legs.

2. Pelvic floor: tighten and relax the muscles around the urethra, vagina, and anus (see also the section below on incontinence).

3. Lie flat on your back with your knees bent up and your feet flat on the surface of the bed or floor; flatten the hollow of your back, hold for a count of five, and then gently relax.

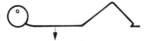

And on the second or third day:

4. Lie flat on your back on a firm surface and stretch one leg away from you while shortening the other—repeat in the opposite direction.

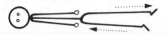

5. Lie as for exercise 3. Stretch your arms out sideways, then lift one arm over your body to touch your hands together. Repeat, rolling in the opposite direction, keeping your knees upright but letting your head move to face the moving arm as you twist at the waist. If your breasts are tender you may like to leave this exercise for a day or two.

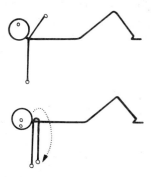

6. Lie as for exercise 5. Contract your abdominal muscles, keep your arms still, and move your legs (knees together) slowly to one side. Come up again, relax, and then repeat to the other side. Feel the pull of the muscles as the legs go down towards the bed.

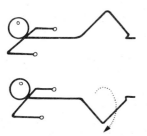

7a. Lie as for exercise 3, contract your abdominal muscles, and lift your head to look at your knees. Pressing your elbows on the bed can help you.

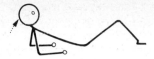

7b. As your muscles get stronger, do this exercise raising your hands to touch your knees.

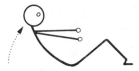

NB   Do not do this last exercise with straight legs and your toes hooked under furniture—it can damage your back—and always lift your head and shoulders towards your feet, not both legs in the air towards your head.

Each exercise may be repeated five to ten times daily and the difficulty increased not only by the number of times of repetition but also by the speed with which you perform the exercises—the slower the movement the harder your muscles have to work, especially in exercise 7.

After a general anaesthetic

Breathing exercises are necessary. Sit or lie in a comfortable position, sigh a long breath out, refill your lungs, and blow out so that you feel that your ribs are like fingers squeezing out the spongy tissue of your lungs. Repeat this 10 times two or three times a day. If you have had a Caesarean section you will be more comfortable if you support the scar with your hands while doing the deep breathing and if you need to cough. Do what you can of exercises 1–7 above, but only within the limits of pain.

Getting out of bed

Before you start to walk, correct your posture. Your centre of gravity will have changed now your baby is born and you may feel strangely 'empty' and exposed without a 'bump' in front. Stand tall, feet slightly apart, and gently rock from heel to toe. When you feel comfortably balanced, move carefully. This is particularly important if you have stitches as there is an automatic tendency to hunch yourself forward—if you have abdominal stitches this will cause the weight of the internal organs to fall forward against the scar and make it more painful. If you aim to push the top of your head forward and up this will straighten your spine, you can relax your shoulders, and a lot of your 'spare tyre' will disappear. Standing correctly is good exercise for your abdominal and back muscles—so check frequently on your posture.

Backache

This may result from a variety of causes, for example from bad posture during pregnancy, an epidural anaesthetic, changing the baby's nappy at a height that means you have to stoop, from pushing a pram, carry-cot, etc. with a handle that is not the right height for you, and so on. Your first objective is to get rid of the cause of the trouble if possible—maybe shoes with a different height of heel will help or a different surface on which to handle the baby, or being careful how you lift the baby, carry shopping, etc. If you use a baby sling, check that you stand straight and do not carry a baby who is too heavy for you, even if the sling is sufficiently strong.

While the backache is severe, try lying flat on the floor on your back, perhaps with your head raised about a centimetre (could be on a magazine). Gently stretch your arms and legs, let them relax, and feel the firm, level surface beneath you. Rest like this as often as you can—perhaps sometimes with your feet raised as well. Gradually progressing to 'sit-ups' as in exercise 7 above will also help to get rid of the backache. An exercise called 'high dog crawl' can also help backache: kneel on all fours, (a) bend up one knee to touch your forehead (you will need to drop your head to reach) and then (b) stretch your leg out straight behind you and raise your head. Repeat with alternate legs. Correct your posture whatever position you are in, making sure that if you are sitting your back is fully supported. Once you have had your postnatal check, swimming—especially breast-stroke—is very good for your back and your whole body, and you may like to ask your doctor's advice on taking up other forms of exercise.

Prolapse of the uterus and stress incontinence

A prolapsed uterus is one which has slipped downwards. Slackness of the pelvic floor muscles is usually the root cause of prolapse and stress incontinence (leaking urine on exertion). The three main aids to correcting these tiresome conditions are:

1. Correct diet—being overweight and being constipated are bad.

2. Correct posture—preferably avoiding standing still.

3. Exercise: the following exercises may be performed sitting well back on a hard chair (or perhaps on the lavatory, although not for prolonged periods), leaning forward, elbows on knees, *or* lying on your back with your knees bent up and your feet flat on the floor or with your legs up and supported against the wall or on a low chair.

(a) Pull up the whole pelvic floor (the area between your legs), hold it tight, aiming at a count of five, and then gently let go.

(b) See if you can isolate the muscle areas—imagining you want to spend a penny and have to wait—concentrate on the muscles round the urethra and tighten them (you can practise 'stream-stopping' on the lavatory)—then tighten the anus, then thirdly pull the vagina up inside you, hold it tight for a count of five, then gently let it down again and finish by slightly tightening.

These movements may be progressed by doing them in a standing position and should be practised in bed before you get up in the morning as well as frequently during the day—increasing to about 100 contractions spread in groups of ten over the day. Get into the habit of doing them whilst you clean your teeth, wash up, wait for the kettle to boil, stand in a queue, etc. They can also be done on all fours, combined with humping and hollowing the lower back. If you have a cough or cold, consciously tighten the pelvic floor before coughing or sneezing; and always remember that checking your posture should include tightening the sling of pelvic muscles to guard the openings in it. Homoeopathic sepia can help to tone slack muscles and thus aid the prevention of 'dribbling' urine on exertion, and also help to aid a prolapse to return to normal; but do consult your doctor if you think you have any bladder or uterus problems.

Many women find they are 'leaky' after childbirth, but nearly always this can be cleared up without the need for an operation; however, *regular* tightening of the muscles is essential, in particular remembering to tighten them before you lift anything, or if you are running, jumping, or doing any other exercise. Once you can control the pelvic floor when you are sitting or standing still, you can learn to do it when you are moving. *Empty your bladder first:*

1. Tighten your pelvic floor muscles and then run on the spot—for as long as you can manage.

2. Jump with both feet together—repeat bouncing jumps for as long as you can manage.

3. Stride jumps—jump your feet apart, together, and so on.

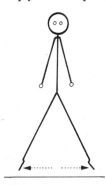

4. Star jumps, as in exercise 3, but as you jump apart, fling your arms up to '10 to 2', and drop them to your sides as you

close your feet. Having mastered these with an empty bladder, try them without emptying your bladder first. If you can manage to do these exercises with a full bladder your muscles will be totally reliable.

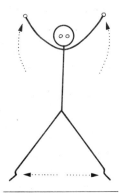

Small disposable absorbent pads may be worn as an interim measure, but don't get into the trap of relying on these instead of doing your exercises: *the problem will not clear up by itself*.

Postnatal support

In providing services to support the mother with a new baby, The National Childbirth Trust does not imply that everyone will need—or wish—to make use of them. If you are in good health, with a thriving and contented baby, and comfortably settled in your home, with friends and family near at hand, you may well feel that life has never been better! You may welcome the release from the routines of your former employment and, despite the ceaseless round of feeding and washing that babies entail, find great pleasure not only in your baby but in a variety of home-based activities for which you had little leisure when you were out at work. You may, or may not, wish to take advantage of the additional contact available through NCT postnatal support groups, where your calmness and general *joie de vivre* may be a great help to those who are lonely or experiencing problems.

Alas, not everyone finds life with a new baby so congenial. The subject of crying babies is one which is often aired in mothers' groups. Especially with a first baby, the reality of how much attention a baby requires can be very different from the parents' expectations. It can be distressing if your baby seems to be asking for help and you don't know what to do. The practical problems are the more obvious ones of hunger, the need to be cuddled, or to be wrapped more warmly. With a less obvious solution are problems caused by, for instance, a difficult birth. This may provide you with a definite answer to people who seem to imply that you are not being a 'good' mother—and as the baby matures he will gradually grow out of his distress.

The baby's crying is his only means of verbal communication, so unless you are really desperate and can't trust yourself not to harm the baby, don't ignore him when he wants you. Imagine how you would feel if you were really upset and needing help and nobody could be bothered with you. Offer him the solace of crying in your arms, held against your face or chest, for as long as you feel able. However, you must be honest with yourself and acknowledge if you have reached the end of your tether. You should then put him safely in his own bed and go away till you feel better.

At an NCT postnatal support group you may well find a multitude of answers to problems with a crying baby, but probably the greatest comfort will be in sharing your worries with people who understand.

Not infrequently, the birth of her first baby heralds a time of great loneliness for a woman. Couples may move to a new home in another district when they start a family; while others have had limited opportunity to make friends in their neighbourhood, when they were both out at work all day. Babies (lovable though they may be) cannot compensate for the variety of stimuli provided by, say, a day at the office, and chatting about the weather with the girl at the cash desk of the supermarket is a poor exchange for sharing daily life with friends and colleagues who really know and appreciate you. NCT postnatal support may be particularly helpful in this kind of situation.

Friendly support

The opportunity to meet other mothers with babies over a cup of coffee is offered by the NCT in many areas, to help the new mother overcome her loneliness and make new friends. These gatherings are usually held in members' homes, weekly, fortnightly, or monthly. If you have attended NCT antenatal classes you will be informed if such arrangements exist in your own locality, but such get-togethers (unless they are specifically 'class reunions') are open to any new mother who, having contacted her local Branch or Group to find out time and place, can be assured of a warm welcome. Additional social activities are organized in many parts of the country and such mutual services as baby-sitting clubs have proved very popular.

Most Branches and Groups produce regular newsletters with articles of interest to parents of a baby or toddler, and valuable information about local services such as the facilities offered in shops and public places for feeding and changing babies, sports facilities for mothers with young families, and mother and toddler clubs. In fact, NCT members prove a mine of information on everything that concerns the new mother, from knitting patterns to the current local rate for baby-minders if you are to return to work. Some Branches have specialist groups (such as Caesarean, miscarriage, single-parent families, working mothers) or they keep a list of people to contact on a one-to-one basis in case of handicap or other problems.

Help in a crisis

The best laid plans for joyful parenthood can be upset by a sudden crisis on the domestic front. In any part of the country where there are NCT members, you can expect to find people who are responsive to your needs when an emergency arises, and in a number of larger Branches and Groups a postnatal support secretary can call upon volunteers who are organized to give help in a crisis. For instance, a 'milk run' may be set up for a mother who is expressing breast milk for her hospitalized baby, or a 'chauffeur' provided for someone who has to keep hospital appointments but is unfit to drive or travel on public transport. Not infrequently, a mother who is unwell may welcome temporary assistance with shopping and household chores, or with ferrying another child to nursery school or play group. Postnatal support 'helpers' may come into antenatal classes to explain the services offered and may, in addition, call in when you and the baby are home from hospital, as a reminder that they are there to hand if needed. However, all such postnatal services are organized on a local basis so there is no uniform pattern, and often no great degree of formality in the arrangements, which are, after all, only an extended form of good-neighbourliness.

In the early months, the majority of mothers experience at least some moments of depression, anxiety or extreme fatigue; for some the condition may be severe and long-lasting. At such a time it is hard to be outgoing and to participate in such events as coffee mornings for new mothers, when it may require a superhuman effort merely to face the daily round. If you feel like this, you may find yourself shunning the company even of old friends and neighbours, especially if you sense their criticism of your apparent lethargy and inability to cope domestically. You may find comfort, at such a time, in the friendship of an NCT member who has perhaps herself had personal experience of postnatal depression, or has the personal qualities necessary to accept you, just as you are, in your present unhappiness.

In some situations there is of course every reason for distress. A baby may be sick, sometimes dying, or born with a handicap, in which case practical as well as emotional assistance may be required. However hard it may be for you to talk about your anxiety and grief, you should be able to expect from NCT members compassion and a readiness to be available when needed, to listen and support.

If the NCT is not listed in the local telephone directory, apply to Headquarters and you will be put in touch with an appropriate person.

Although a great deal of this book is directed towards mothers' needs, some groups now have fathers' support groups, and couples' classes are available in many areas.

Postnatal depression

Your baby has been born, you are surrounded by flowers and messages of congratulation—everything should be marvellous. The first couple of days after the birth have been filled with euphoria, now suddenly all you want to do is weep. You are obsessed with small details of your labour, where you feel somehow you failed; every whimper from the baby heralds a disaster; every word from the nurses brings you to the verge of tears.

This describes to some extent how you may feel shortly after the birth of your baby. It is usually called 'the third-day blues' and a large proportion of women experience the feeling. For the majority, it is soon over. However, some women may find that they are engulfed by depression for a time some days after they leave hospital, while a tiny minority experience such severe depression that they need special care.

Depression

Depression can mean different things to different people. For some it is a transient mood, and for others, a lasting emotional experience usually associated with an important event in life. Other people may think of depression as a shameful illness and a breakdown from normality. Perhaps depression can be described best as a part of life, ranging from the mood swings known to most people, to deep despair and mental disorder.

Postnatal depression

When birth is this big event in your life, a number of changes take place: the baby is born, you become a mother, your partner is transformed from lover to father, and a new family begins. These changes can expose you to considerable stress and how you cope depends on a complex interaction of factors. The stress can lead to strong feelings, some recognized, others apparently coming from nowhere. If these feelings become too strong, they get 'switched off' and depression is experienced.

Birth   It is estimated that two-thirds of all women experience some degree of depression after childbirth. There seems some evidence that the birth itself—the quality of your antenatal preparation, the attitudes of your medical attendants, the kind of delivery you have, whether or not the baby is left with you, and how feeding is established—affects how you adapt to these changes, and how you see yourself in the new identity of mother. Yet depression may still occur with the best preparation and birth experience. If your 'baby-blues' are due to overtiredness and mental exhaustion then a couple of days of leaving everything that isn't essential can be the answer. Use disposable nappies, leave the ironing and housework, and, most importantly, have plenty of rest and eat more—avoiding 'junk' foods (artificially treated, flavoured, processed) and eating a nourishing snack or meal about every two-and-a-half to three hours and possibly taking vitamin B6 as a supplement. Ask your doctor's advice about how much you should take, or take complete vitamin B formula, which is correctly balanced. Try to allow some time for yourself: that is a time when you follow a particular interest of your own other than looking after the baby. Don't suddenly drop all the things you liked to do beforehand.

Hormonal causes   During pregnancy, the hormones in your body undergo significant changes in order to enable the baby to grow, to set labour in motion, and to stimulate lactation. For example, progesterone (which, among its functions, is responsible for a feeling of well-being) increases production a hundredfold during pregnancy. This hormone ensures that the baby obtains adequate nourishment through the placenta, which itself becomes an extra production centre. After the birth the placenta is discarded and a rapid drop in the production of progesterone takes place. The hormonal system then lives in a temporary state of imbalance. Many women experience 'blues' in this period, with tears alternating with excitement and awe. These rapid and often bewildering changes of mood may last for a few days, but with loving care, understanding and quiet confidence from your partner and attendants, you may find yourself settling down. The normal production of progesterone begins again as in the non-pregnant state. There are other hormonal influences and further implications of hormonal imbalance are currently being investigated.

Social and physical causes   For other women, the transition takes longer. The new mother leaves hospital with high expectations of herself. Sometimes she has not been married for long, often she may be living far from close friends and family. She may have had a good job in which she felt capable and financially independent. Motherhood seems a difficult role. Her skills no longer work. The baby cries, her partner comes home hungry and tired, she knows nobody to talk with during the day and the organization of time becomes chaotic. She becomes anxious and the baby responds with further crying and unsettled sleep. Physical fatigue sets in—somehow there is never enough time and sleep becomes an all-consuming need. She finds herself longing for old freedoms and for the bliss of the early days of the relationship. She tries again and again to sort it all out, but the secret eludes her. Everyone else seems to be coping: why isn't she? She looks tired and lethargic, and feels a sense of despair and loneliness, of being overwhelmed and losing herself. Sexually, she feels too tired to make love, and then realizes that she does not want to anyway, and takes this as proof of her inadequacy as a woman. She may try to explain to other people, but she may also give up, and retreat into apathetic silences or irritable flare-ups, feeling guilty and unlovable inside. Many men feel upset and bewildered if their partners behave in this way, though some may be able to perceive that the woman has been unable to adjust emotionally and physically to the new role of mother.

If you feel like this, you will probably be in a downward spiral of fatigue and loss of confidence. If your partner can see this and understand, he may be able to shift his own position by helping more, expecting less and showing you that he loves you and has faith in you. He should look for solutions which fit your temperament and needs, perhaps by arranging visits to or from someone, by feeding the baby at night for a week (even with a breastfed baby he can give an occasional bottle), by asking the doctor for sleeping tablets to help you, and by taking extra time off work so that he can help in a practical way and share your knowledge of how demanding a baby can be (most people don't realize how emotionally exhausting it may be to have a crying baby whom you can find no way of soothing). Extra sleeping time and outings together, and on your own without the baby, can help you to feel your way gradually into a more stable position. The anxiety lessens, the baby settles and the transition comes to an end. You can be yourself, *and* a mother, and your expectations are more realistic.

If you need a nanny on a regular basis, apply to your nearest College of Further Education which runs a NNEB course (for nursery nurses) and you may well find a local person who would be very pleased to help you, either a young girl who wants a full-time job, or a mature student wanting occupation which fits in with looking after her own family. For further advice try *The Working Mother's Handbook* (see Further reading, p. 290).

Non-understanding　Resolution of the problem is unfortunately not always so straightforward. Your partner may be genuinely bewildered and respond by telling you to 'pull yourself together', resulting in further tears and distress for you. It seems as if the birth has triggered off memories of old losses and as if you yourself crave the soothing care and attention of a mother. Responsibility becomes a burden and you may find it difficult to share the strength of your feelings, which may be quite horrifying to you. You may even find yourself wishing to harm the baby, which naturally fills you with shame and guilt. Your partner feels powerless. It is difficult for you both to imagine that any other couple could feel so despairing, and you are unable to share the pain with others or with one another. Communications break down.

Treatment

Family and community help   Depression which comes with a 'life event' progresses in a way which tends to be self-healing, and the experience can be a crucial point of growth towards maturity and a clearer picture of yourself and your family. This does not mean that the time of depression is any less painful, nor does it mean that it is a helpful response to say only that it will soon be all over. Active support during a time of depression is still essential. There are resources to help a family through the experience. If you have learned about depression in preparation classes, you can be aware of what is happening. The feelings can be shared and a survival campaign worked out. Preparation classes themselves give a network of supporting friends, and opportunities for postnatal occasions and individual counselling. In many areas The National Childbirth Trust runs classes which continue after the birth, when you return to your former class with your baby, and share your experiences. You are introduced to other mothers in your area, providing friendship and babysitting help. Such self-help groups can be invaluable to young parents (see 'Postnatal support', p. 256). The community itself helps where the wider family is no longer near enough to give practical and physical support.

Professional services   There are professional workers who can be consulted about postnatal depression. The health visitor who comes to see you at home can be sensitively understanding and supportive, with extra visits and practical encouragement. The general practitioner can assess the situation in your whole family. He can prescribe drugs to help you to sleep and may suggest a course of anti-depressant pills. Since an inability to cope is probably one reason for your depression, tranquillizers are not appropriate treatment—you would not be helped much by living in a drugged 'tranquillized' state all day because it would make it difficult to look after yourself and the baby. Sometimes it is hard to find the right kind of help. The health visitor and GP may seem to have little time to listen and explain, and you may trail off apologetically at the end of a wasted visit. In this kind of situation, it can help if your husband is present at the consultation. You will also need to return to your doctor if the prescribed medication proves unsatisfactory. If you can both recognize what is happening and accept that you need help, you can usually find someone to share the problem. This does require a certain amount of courage but sometimes the right person appears in an unexpected guise. The deepest need does seem to be for warm accepting human contact at this time. There is a Social Services Department in every town where help may be available from a social worker. The Samaritan Service, MIND groups, and the Association for Postnatal Illness are other sources of help, and can be found in the telephone directory. Some mothers have found that homoeopathy helped them through this distressing period.

Mental disorder

There are some mothers who go further along the continuum of distress into mental disorder, when they act in unusual ways and become out of touch with reality. In this situation it is important that a doctor is called even without the woman's permission. She may need special care in a hospital, where she can be looked after with her baby until she can take over responsibility for herself again. Depression of this kind may have shown symptoms in earlier life. If this is known, a woman can have skilled therapy before the birth to minimize the subsequent situation and to establish a support system ready to go into action. Progesterone therapy has been shown to be helpful for some women. Psychotherapy after the birth may also be useful.

Prevention

In our present state of knowledge, it would be foolish to think that all depression could be prevented. If depression is part of change and growth, perhaps the task is to accept it with information and understanding. By taking away some of the panic and fear of the unknown, inner resources can be mobilized more easily and sharing can take place. Preparation groups which cover the periods before and after the birth provide information, support and friendly faces as well as practical help. Knowledge of the local services and how to use them is important for all families. For a couple, it is important to establish trustworthy friendships before the birth of the baby if they cannot turn to the wider family, and to know how to contact a counsellor in the community.

The new family

Each new family must work out its own structure and relation-ships: words of advice in a book will make little difference to serious problems and will be unnecessary if everything instinc-tively goes well. However, in the time of change after the birth of a first baby, it can be easy to adopt patterns of behaviour which may cause stress later on, and to slip into habits which are hard to break even when common sense tells you they are harmful. Perhaps what follows may help you to nip such tendencies in the bud.

Family structure

When the new baby arrives he naturally becomes the focus of attention. This is good and inevitable but you should be careful to make sure that the baby does not become *too* important. All the members of your new family are equally valuable: the baby and his needs should fit into the existing family framework wherever possible. Don't change your lifestyle completely just because you are now parents—you are more than likely to come to resent the baby's intrusion into your settled ways. Fit in with his overwhelming needs—feed him when he is hungry, cuddle him when he is lonely, change his nappies when he is smelly. But, having satisfied these basic physical needs, start to satisfy your own while making allowances for his presence. If you want to make a journey, take him with you; if you need a break, leave him with a reliable baby-sitter; if you are invited to a party, take him too if practical. Accustom the child to a life full of new experiences, always buffered by your love and calmness, and you will lay good foundations for later. It is not kind, in the long run, to 'hibernate' for the sake of your young baby. You all miss a lot of fun and sharing.

It is possible to let the pendulum swing too far in the other direction and, instead of the baby being the boss, the parents are not realistic in making allowance for its dependence and needs. Knowing what small babies can and cannot do, and how they develop over the first months, is important. Just as it is not wise to change your entire lifestyle when a baby arrives, it is equally unwise to expect a baby to make no difference at all.

Couples will want to ensure that their own relationship does not get out of balance either. They are not overnight recast as 'the baby's father and mother'. Each will need to be careful not to presume on the other, and an honest sharing of feelings and tasks will make a great difference. At one end of the scale you may have a woman with a gentle doting partner who is so self-indulgent about her vulnerability as a mother that she tricks him into doing everything for her: what starts as constant requests for help can turn, over the months, into a full-blown matriarchy and exploitation of the man's good nature. Heavy-handed patriarchs, at the other end of the scale, are not common nowadays, but if your partner shows this tendency in a way which you feel is damaging to the marriage or to the baby, use your skill and patience to divert him from this role. Couples whose relationship falls somewhere in the middle of these two extremes can still hurt one another thoughtlessly. It is easy to see how difficulties can arise from different viewpoints: the new mother may regard herself as 'being stuck at home all day looking after a demanding baby' and feel she deserves some looking after by her partner when he comes home—whereas he may feel he is quite justified in expecting meals ready without fail because she has 'nothing to do all day except look after a little baby'.

Sometimes a couple's longed-for baby becomes so precious to them that in their eyes he changes from an ordinary little human being into a love object. He ceases to be a person, with mortal qualities and faults, and is a little idol whom they worship for their own gratification. Every need or imagined whim is indulged by the adoring parents, and the child becomes a greedy monster destined either for a later rude awakening or for lifelong unpopularity with his fellows. Because he is not treated like an ordinary person, the child misses the rough and tumble of normal growing-up and his grip on the world is unsound. The parents of such a child never really get to know him, either because they project all their fantasies on to him, or because they are so interested in their own feelings that they do not bother about his. For all concerned, the creation of a love object is unhealthy.

In an ideal world everyone would know their partner so well that they would be able to predict how parenthood would affect them; but we don't always anticipate our own reactions, far less those of our partners. It should not be taken for granted that women will be transformed overnight into Mother Earth figures who can instinctively feed, pacify, and cherish a squalling newborn child. By the same token, it should not be assumed that fathers will be bowled over by the minutiae of babyhood—nappies, feeds, and achievements—to the exclusion of everything else. There is more to life than nappy pails, but the woman who is too harrassed to realize this is in danger of neglecting her relationship. Equally the man who disregards these matters, denying the importance of being a mother, also puts the relationship under stress.

Changing perspectives

Most parents, expectant or fulfilled, find that their ideas of entertainment and leisure-time pursuits change as they get used to thinking of themselves as a family with children instead of just a couple, so that far from grumbling about not being able to be as they were before, they are delighted to move into a new era in their lives and to share its pleasures and compensations. Pregnancy and labour are great adventures, and parenthood progresses slowly enough to allow for gradual adaptation and immense pleasure not only in guiding the development and interests of your child but also in seeing the world afresh through his eyes.

Sharing

Share the babycare tasks which can be divided between you, but do this because you want equal loving contact with the baby and not because they are chores. Be realistic about sharing. In coping with night feeds, for instance, your husband may happily help by picking up the baby, but he need not be forced to share your broken nights if it makes difficulties: he cannot catnap at work, during the day, to make up the sleep deficit. He can make his contribution at another time, by helping with the housework, cuddling or bathing the baby, or changing nappies. Work out what suits you both best and enjoy your baby together.

Some people still think that babycare is 'woman's work' and this can cause problems. It may be that the new mother gets pleasure from feeling indispensable, or that she has old-fashioned ideas about gender roles. By monopolizing the baby she can frustrate her partner's desire to be a tender and caring father, and can hurt him very much. On the other hand, a new father may leave the children entirely to the mother, thus cutting himself off from them and from her. Parenthood is basically begun as a shared thing and should continue that way.

Some parents may decide on a more radical division of child care, or feel that in their case it is more appropriate that the mother goes to work and the father looks after the child(ren). It can prove difficult to break the traditional role-pattern established in one's own childhood, not only domestically but also in relation to the world outside. A man may feel ill at ease using facilities for children where the attending adults are usually women (for example play groups); when taking a child out the poor provision of social facilities can become all too evident as the need to change a nappy develops into a major problem. A mother may be surprised to find how jealous she feels when the baby starts to respond more easily to its father, or the father becomes better at interpreting the infant's signals. (The same situation can arise with baby-minders.)

Sharing the caring, if both parents are happy with their roles, can have long-term benefits in that both will be alert to the child's physical and emotional needs and understanding of the difficulties arising. The burden of sole responsibility is relieved.

First-time parents should recognize that a significant proportion of their practical childcare techniques derives from how they themselves were brought up. It can be unsettling for two people who are perfectly happily married to discover how different these background experiences can be. You are well advised to talk with each other about this so that you don't unconsciously cause unnecessary strains by working on different assumptions. It is astonishing to discover the heated arguments which can arise over how to fold and fasten a nappy. The tiniest matters will come under scrutiny, and probably won't show until mother, father, and baby are all at home at the same time. Then you realize the incredible variety of theories on child care and that the way your family did things was only one of many approaches.

If you as a couple have faced some of these choices, laughed at their seeming importance and begun to set your own ways of caring for your own baby, you will be off to a good start and will not be upset by people advising yet another approach.

Confidence

Have confidence in the way you handle your baby. He is part of you both, and you soon know him better than anyone else does. Once you have decided on a rough 'philosophy' for bringing up your child, support one another in it. Be true to your own convictions and don't feel bound by fashion or by family traditions.

Be patient with those who want to help you. The company of new parents, however confident and accomplished they are, brings out both the protective and the bossy instincts in other couples. You will never be at a loss for advice. Be tolerant and remember that you, in turn, will be tempted to treat other new parents in exactly the same way!

Your parents and older relatives will feel especially responsible for you and it may require almost superhuman efforts on their behalf not to bombard you with their worries and reminiscences. They may have unrealistically rosy ideas about how well they coped with you as a new baby. Respect their experience as parents (after all, you have thrived!) while treating their advice in the light of your own beliefs. Do not allow anyone to destroy your confidence in what you think is best, but be prepared to learn from all available sources. Remember, as far as childcare fashions go, there is nothing new under the sun.

The new baby and the toddler

When you are expecting a baby and there is already at least one older child in the family the most common worry is the possible jealousy which might be shown by the older siblings. There are certain ways you can prepare your children for the arrival of a new baby. Displacement is inevitable—jealousy is not necessarily automatic and can be minimized if it does occur. You can discuss the arrival of the new baby by using books to help interest the child (list available from NCT Education Committee). You should warn the toddler that the baby will not be a playmate in the beginning. Using photographs of your other children when newborn babies may help them to think of the differences whilst reminding them that they too were once so tiny and helpless. Seeing someone else's new baby will help with this aspect too.

Remember your toddler was a baby himself very recently and don't expect him to grow up too abruptly. This is not the best time to start toilet training, play group, etc.; either before or afterwards would be better. If he regresses, try to accept this without comment. It will pass. After all, the baby does wet his pants all the time and you're not cross with him . . .

Assure the toddler he will still be able to do the things he likes doing (play group, swimming, visiting friends, having friends to play) and be sure you do what you promise.

It is unlikely that your child will see the baby at birth, more likely that he will see the baby for the first time when he visits you in hospital. If his first view of the baby is of it in your arms, cuddle the toddler as well and then introduce him to the baby. Try not to let other visitors ignore him in favour of the baby.

If the toddler is to move into a different room, move him well in advance of the baby arriving and make his new bedroom an exciting place to be in. If the toddler likes sleeping in the cot, rather than making him give it up, it may be worth buying a second one or borrowing one to tide you over the time when you need two cots.

Reassure the toddler about his new position in the family. You may wish to give him a present when you come home from hospital—but don't tell him the baby brought it—that's not true! If you show the toddler you love him and the baby, the toddler will follow your example and feel himself secure also. If you give the toddler the impression that the baby is a nuisance, he is likely to hurt it—to try to get rid of it for you. Help him to express what he is feeling and show him love and understanding. He still needs as much as he was getting before the baby arrived. A second baby cannot have the same amount of company from you as the first but what he loses from you he gains from the older children, and this can more than make up for the lack of time you have available.

Very young children have natural abilities in the way they handle babies. Do give them the chance to hold the baby—they will probably naturally support the head. Let your toddler help look after the baby by fetching nappies, creams, etc., but do not overdo the 'little helper' aspect—it can pall very quickly.

Your toddler can no longer have you to himself; your relationship must change. Instead of him being totally dependent on you, show him that you need his support and friendship. Most toddlers will be proud and pleased to be needed so much. If you try to exclude the toddler or older children from your new relationship with the baby, that is when the problems start. Aggression may be diverted at the mother or other children with whom he plays, or his toys. Stop him from causing hurt or damage, but don't get cross.

Also remember that babies, as you will have learned already, can put up with a lot of physical attention. The older child's play behaviour with the baby can look very rough, but it is these games the baby loves and as long as you are there to keep an eye on things it can be rewarding for toddler and baby. However, do be careful where the baby is left when you are not in the room. Never leave the baby in a bouncing cradle or relax-chair on a table or work-top because the toddler may accidentally pull him off. The floor is much safer. It may be a good idea to put the carry-cot inside a dropside cot rather than on a stand which might be pulled over.

Children are naturally good with babies and are often marvellously loving and tolerant. Trust them! They will, however, need to 'escape' at times from the youngster. Make sure they have private space, and that their treasures are out of the baby's reach. A play-pen is often more useful to a pre-school child who is drawing and trying to keep his efforts from being spoiled than it is to a crawling baby.

Older children

If you have an older child, you can discuss his feelings with him. Warn him that there may well be times when he thinks the baby is a nuisance and reassure him that this is perfectly reasonable. If he can tell you about it at the time it may be possible to help him come to terms with the situation; it may also make you realize that you are shutting out the older child from your attention. It should never be made necessary for him to give up his special interests because there is a new baby in the family.

Improvising

Don't try to keep up with the Joneses if you can't afford to. Set a fashion for self-help and eccentricity by buying second-hand equipment (wash it thoroughly before use), the minimum number of baby clothes (you may receive a lot as presents), and by spending your money on items like high quality terry nappies (or disposable ones, if you prefer), which will save time and effort later. If, as a housewife, you totter from one muddle to the next, it may be better to spend the Child Benefit Allowance on once-a-week domestic help rather than on a succession of baby-suits or as a supplement to the housekeeping funds.

Whole industries are created when manufacturers invent a 'need' for the babycare market. Take heart that the human race has survived until now with these 'needs' unsatisfied. Use your ingenuity for making labour-saving items. The possibilities for improvisation are endless: though safety must always be the prime factor in any do-it-yourself designs.

Resist impulse buys for the child and don't spend a lot of money on toys. Your baby is blissfully unaware of his material status—all he cares about is your loving, consistent care.

And finally . . .

If for any reason your actual birth experience did not come up to your expectation, or you can't (or don't want to) breastfeed, it is unnecessary to feel guilty about it. You have not been responsible for what has happened, so guilt is quite out of place. To feel guilty about having needed medical technology and expertise during your labour is to deny the progress in obstetrics and paediatrics which has taken place in the last generation. And to feel guilty if you are repelled by the thought of breastfeeding your baby is wrong too.

Events rarely go according to the mental plan you conjure up beforehand. Your experiences in pregnancy, labour, and child-care, will inevitably turn out to be different from your anticipations. What matters is how you deal with the real experiences. Don't waste time and emotional energy feeling guilty or disappointed about the failure of your fantasies to stand up to reality.

Preparing for pregnancy

This may seem to be the wrong end of the book for such a chapter, but we have to assume that you purchased the book because you were already pregnant and we know that many people think of this aspect only before a second or later pregnancy. All the information does of course relate to thinking about a first pregnancy also. Remember that it is never too late to help your baby by such actions as improving your diet or stopping smoking. The information and suggestions given here are for you to place alongside all the other considerations which affect your life as you make your decisions about when to have your children.

Nearly every woman wonders if the baby growing inside her will be all right. We may have no control over averting some forms of handicap, but by acting positively we can try to lessen the risks. By the time you are eight weeks pregnant the baby's organs have formed. It is during these first weeks that the baby is at its most vulnerable: a time when many people don't know, or are just beginning to realize, that they are pregnant. So think ahead, say at least four months ahead.

Good food

Taking care over the food both you and your partner eat is one of the best things you can do to improve the health of the future mother and father. As well as providing you with what you need nutritionally, good food can protect you from harmful substances. Even though you may feel fine your developing baby can be affected in the early weeks if just one vital ingredient is missing from the diet. (Most cell formation needs between 30 and 60 nutrients present in appropriate amounts.)

So what should you do? You can move over to the healthier things already in your diet, and reduce as much as possible the processed, manufactured foods, especially those containing sugar, refined (white) flour, food additives (particularly colour and preservatives). Become a label reader. Notice any change in your tastes and respect them.

Best age

Statistics show that the best time to have a baby is in your twenties. If she is younger, a woman may not have finished growing herself. Pregnancy puts additional strain on her resources. As she grows older there is an increased risk of complications and of having a mongol baby (Down's syndrome). Although there is no need to overrate these risks either, taking positive health measures could help to balance any disadvantage.

Birth spacing

Your body needs time to recover after nourishing you and your baby for nine months. If you have had a baby recently it is best to wait about eighteen months before trying to start a new pregnancy, but the emotional well-being of siblings needs consideration too.

After a miscarriage

It may seem hard advice but you will give yourself a real advantage if you wait six months to a year after a miscarriage before starting again. The later the miscarriage, the longer the recovery time needed. This time need not be wasted time: you can plan to use it constructively. This won't make up for losing your baby, but you may find a change in your pace of life is in itself beneficial.

Get to know yourself

The time of preparation for pregnancy is a good time to 'get in touch with your body'. Study its functions, follow your cycles, your ups and downs. Consider which foods taste good to you, what makes you feel lively or low and what helps to release tension so that you can unwind at the end of a day. Your discoveries will be useful to you at all times, especially during pregnancy. Learning to understand and respond to the messages of your body also means you can come to trust your instincts.

Smoking

Smoking is bad for your health but it can be dangerous for your baby too. Perhaps this is the incentive you have always needed to give up. In men fertility can be reduced and sperm damaged by smoking and alcohol. It can increase your risk of miscarriage. It also reduces the nourishment and oxygen a baby receives, leading to smaller babies. Small babies have more problems at birth than others and can be more prone to infection and allergy later.

Drinking

Alcohol has lots of calories but little food value and may interfere with the way the body uses vitamins and minerals essential for your baby's growth. There seems to be no amount which can be said to be altogether 'safe'. Babies born to alcoholic mothers can suffer from 'fetal alcohol syndrome' and have severe defects.

Pollution

As far as possible, avoid the everyday things which contain poison: traffic fumes, lead, chemicals at work, DDT and other pesticides (including household fly-killers), X-rays and radiation. Dodging these things is not always easy, so remember the protective effect of eating well.

Slimming

If you are thinking of having a baby, this is not the time to go on a slimming diet. Not only can it reduce your fertility, but it can make you more subject to producing an abnormal child. If you are considerably overweight, consult a dietitian, but do not try to get to a 'fashionable' weight at this time. You may find a change to a healthy wholefood diet—high in fibre, low in sugar, and moderate in fat—helps anyway.

The pill

If you have been using a contraceptive pill, come off it at least four months before trying to conceive and use an alternative form of contraception meanwhile. Even the low-dosage contraceptive pills interfere with the way the body uses vitamins and minerals and alter your hormonal balance; so give your body time to get back to normal (at least three and preferably five periods).

Medicines

If consulting your doctor at this time, tell him you are hoping to become pregnant; this will ensure that any medicines prescribed will be safe. If you can, avoid taking any medicines, for example sleeping-pills or even aspirin. Try other methods of getting to sleep, like relaxation. Learn to practise this technique in the period of preparation for pregnancy.

Vaginal discharge

If you are not happy about any vaginal discharge, consult your GP. As sexually transmitted diseases seem to be on the increase, it is wise to check and get anything treated, if necessary, before you become pregnant.

German measles

Protect yourself against German measles (rubella). A mild illness for you, if can be disastrous for the baby if caught in the first four months of pregnancy. It is worth while asking your GP to check if you have antibodies to the disease. If not, one injection will give protection (you should check to make sure it has taken) but you must avoid becoming pregnant during the following three months.

Problems in the family

If a relative has had a baby with a defect, you may ask your GP to refer you to a genetic counsellor. You can then discuss the chances of your baby having a similar problem. Ask what action you can take to lessen any risks. The advice given in this section should be of help.

Your general health

Before you become pregnant, aim to clear up any minor ailments or other health problems you may suffer from: nagging coughs, persistent colds, headaches, or skin problems. A good diet with plenty of fresh fruit and vegetables and wholegrain products, along with exercise and fresh air, will help, but if you still don't feel at your best consult your doctor with a view to getting rid of any remaining problems. If your problem is a bad back, it could get worse in pregnancy, so consider now your posture and the way you lift things and carry them.

All these suggestions should help you to become fitter and should be of benefit in the long run too when you find yourself coping with a new baby.

Introducing The National Childbirth Trust (NCT)

Our organization was founded in 1956 to improve women's knowledge about childbirth and to promote the teaching of relaxation and breathing for labour. In the years of experience since then, we have learned from mothers of other needs surrounding the experience of pregnancy and parenthood, there have been major changes in hospital routines and procedures, and we have widened our interests, the scope of our literature, and our training courses in response.

The NCT is a growing and flexible organization, maintaining its primary interest in the importance of excellent antenatal preparation. Members come from all walks of life—professional, skilled, unskilled—and each offers particular knowledge which is relevant to the field of early parenthood. NCT work overlaps into many specialities: teaching, obstetrics, paediatrics, social work, and psychology, to name but a few. The NCT has advisers from many fields and is continually learning from them: a number of the advisers have contributed to sections in this book. We have found that the value of a multi-disciplinary organization cannot be overestimated in the field of parenthood.

Aims

The National Childbirth Trust aims to set and maintain high standards of antenatal education; to assess the needs of expectant mothers and new parents and to help to get these needs met; to press for informed choice in pregnancy and labour for expectant parents; and to emphasize the need for good emotional support for women in labour.

Antenatal classes

When the NCT was founded, few books about childbirth were available, little encouragement was offered to mothers by the medical profession, and women who asked questions about physical changes during pregnancy and birth were often regarded as unnecessarily inquisitive or over-anxious. The NCT can claim to have had considerable influence in changing this attitude, so that now the woman who wishes to take the trouble to prepare herself to co-operate effectively both with her attendants and with her own body when she is giving birth will usually receive help and encouragement.

NCT antenatal classes are designed to give accurate information enabling prospective parents to understand the natural birth process and how to adapt to difficulties should they arise, and to appreciate when medical intervention is necessary. Through informal discussion parents are helped to consider their own expectations of birth and parenthood; they are encouraged to ask for explanations during antenatal classes and in their contacts with hospital personnel, and to accept that personal responsibility in parenthood starts before birth.

Antenatal teachers and antenatal classes

Education offered to expectant parents should be relevant to their needs. The skill with which this is done will depend largely on the personality, ability, and training of the teacher. So one of our most important aims has been to devise a careful, comprehensive, and stimulating course of teacher training, based on a tutorial system, and to present it in such a way that it can be taken by women who are primarily occupied in bringing up their own children. They know what it feels like to be pregnant and to give birth, but they have learned to listen as well as to teach. Antenatal classes are always informal, with opportunities for discussion as an integral part. Teachers, after their initial training, are provided with a study programme, frequent contact with other teachers who have between them a wide variety of professional and other background knowledge, and they are kept in touch with new ideas in education and in obstetric theory and practice.

Breastfeeding counselling

Breastfeeding has so many advantages for both mother and baby that we actively encourage mothers to choose this method of feeding whenever possible. More and more mothers are choosing to breastfeed, but many give up after a few weeks—although they could almost certainly have continued for longer with the support of an NCT breastfeeding counsellor. Our breastfeeding counsellors have breastfed their own babies and are trained to help and support mothers to achieve and continue breastfeeding. There are nearly 500 breastfeeding counsellors throughout the country, who work on a mother-to-mother basis, as well as promoting breastfeeding in hospitals and schools and at antenatal classes. Many counsellors also fit and sell the unique Mava maternity and nursing bra, designed to adapt to the changes in pregnancy and breastfeeding. Some counsellors hire out electric breast pumps to mothers who need them and also arrange breast-milk collection for milk banks.

Postnatal support

The NCT's support network is on a mother-to-mother, or sometimes parent-to-parent, basis. Any advice given is based on experience with our own children, not on training, assuming that those who have coped with some of the common difficulties which arise in early parenthood are the right people to support new parents faced with similar anxieties. We can't teach people how to be parents, but often our sympathetic 'befrienders' are seen as 'models' who have so far successfully brought up their own children. The most important aspects of this support are that it reinforces the parents' confidence in their ability to care for, and enjoy, their baby, and that it eases the feeling of isolation felt sometimes by new mothers at home alone with their babies. With problems of a serious type, the help we provide is of a facilitating nature—finding for parents the extra help they need, whether it is from professional health workers or from voluntary organizations or self-help groups. There is, of course, often supportive work which Trust members can undertake alongside this. Much of the best support, apart from that given by the family, existing friends, and professional health workers, comes from informal relationships between parents who meet at an antenatal class, clinic, or in hospital, and find they have a great deal in common. Most NCT branches and groups supplement this with more formal schemes to ensure that every new mother is included.

Education in schools

The NCT's experience with thousands of young parents has made us concerned about the lack of information about 'human reproduction', 'child care', and 'preparation for parenthood' given within our educational system. Although relevant subjects are now becoming available in our schools, they tend to be taken up by non-academic girls. Sadly, therefore, these courses remain very much the poor relation of the school curriculum. Many NCT branches have been invited to help with such courses. They make a real-life contribution by organizing visits by mothers (sometimes fathers) with young children and babies to the schools. Pregnancy, birth, breastfeeding, and parenthood are all aspects which might be discussed on such visits. The Education Committee is able to collect and collate information and to co-operate with NCT branches and groups in order to learn from young parents what they wish they had known before they had their babies and hence to organize the NCT's contribution to schools. Anyone embarking on a school programme is welcome to write to the NCT's Education Committee for guidance and lists of resources.

Study events, conferences, and study groups

The NCT holds frequent study days and weekend seminars on many aspects of education for childbirth, parenthood, and breastfeeding. From time to time internationally-known experts are featured at special lectures and study days. Regional conferences, small conferences for specialist groups, and NCT branch conferences are also held. Interdisciplinary groups are convened to study particular aspects of childbirth, and may publish papers on the basis of their discussions. The Trust also runs study days specially designed for midwives and health visitors.

Publications and other services

The NCT has produced a series of leaflets on many aspects of pregnancy, birth, and early parenthood, all of which are revised periodically to keep them up to date. A stock of recommended books is also held and a list is available.

NCT (Maternity Sales) Ltd. markets the unique Mava maternity and nursing brassière, carefully designed in a wide range of sizes to meet the needs of pregnant and nursing mothers. Other products, for parents and babies, are also available. Whilst offering what it hopes are products of service to expectant mothers and new parents, the sales company exists to support the Trust, to whom it covenants its profits. A request for the sales catalogue will also bring you the list of NCT publications and recommended books. NCT (Maternity Sales) Ltd. shares the same address as the Trust (see below).

A hire service for electric breast pumps is organized by NCT branches to help mothers of sick or premature babies to provide breast milk.

Local branches of the NCT in most parts of the United Kingdom offer antenatal classes, breastfeeding counselling, and postnatal support. Try your local telephone directory for a contact.

Otherwise, for details of local representatives, publications, or any of our services, please apply to the NCT as below; postage stamps are always appreciated (please err on the generous side with size of envelope if sending an s.a.e.).

The National Childbirth Trust,
 9 Queensborough Terrace,
 London W2 3TB
 Telephone: 01–221–3833

Homoeopathy

An increasing amount of interest in homoeopathic remedies has been shown in recent years and there are several of these which are reported as having been found of help during pregnancy, labour, and the breastfeeding period: for example, remedies for pregnancy sickness, heartburn, thrush, bruising to the mother and shock to the baby during labour, shortening the labour, speeding the healing of the pelvic floor tissue, breastfeeding problems such as cracked nipples and inflammation of the breasts, the baby's intolerance of diet. Some mothers have found help from homoeopathy whilst living through postnatal depression.

The principle of homoeopathy is treating like with like: a substance which, in its natural state, can create signs of illness in the healthy can, in extreme dilution, promote health in the sick. No harmful side-effects have been observed in over two hundred years of documentation, using the lower potencies as first-aid remedies, and the higher ones with medical supervision. Homoeopathy can combine well with orthodox medicine for treatment in many cases: the treatment is recognized by the DHSS and is available free on the NHS to patients using a medically qualified homoeopathic practitioner or a homoeopathic hospital or out-patients clinic. There are lay homoeopaths, some of whom may be good at prescribing, but as they have no medical qualification and no access to X-rays, pathology laboratories, etc. they may fail to diagnose illness correctly. In cases of illness it is important to get a diagnosis from a doctor so that the appropriate treatment is given.

For further information (book lists, details of stockists of the remedies, and names and addresses of homoeopathic doctors), contact the British Homoeopathic Association, 27a Devonshire Street, London W1 (01–935–2163).

Useful addresses

Within the text of the book we referred to the Vegetarian Society and the Vegan Society. We have the following addresses:

The Vegetarian Society, Parkdale, Durham Road, Altrincham, Cheshire.

The London Vegetarian Centre, 53 Marloes Road, London W8 61D.

The Vegan Society, 47 Highlands Road, Leatherhead, Surrey.

Here is a small selection of other organizations which you or someone you know may wish at some time to contact:

Down's Children's Association (which promotes the care, nurture, and education of persons having Down's syndrome (mongolism), particularly in the early years of life), Quinborne Community Centre, Quinton, Birmingham B32 2T (021–427–1374), and 4 Oxford Street (entrance through Hornes), London W1N 9FL (01–580–0511/2).

Foresight—The Association for the Promotion of Pre-conceptual Care (for help and advice—for instance on nutrition and protection from pollution—to prospective parents), The Old Vicarage, Church Lane, Witley, Surrey GU8 5PN. [Send large s.a.e.]

The Foundation for the Study of Infant Deaths (for information on the sudden infant death syndrome or 'cot deaths'), 5th Floor, 4/5 Grosvenor Place, London SW1 (01–235–1721/01–245–9421). [Send large s.a.e.]

Gingerbread (an association for one-parent families), 35 Wellington Street, London WC2. [Send s.a.e.]

The Miscarriage Association (for support, help, and information), send s.a.e. to Charlotte Gilroy, 2 West Vale, Thornhill Road, Dewsbury, West Yorkshire (0532–828946).

The National Association for the Welfare of Children in Hospital (for information and practical help), Argyle House, 29–31 Euston

Road, London NW1 2SD. [Send s.a.e. for details of local groups.]

Nurture (support for disabled parents). For information contact The National Childbirth Trust at the address quoted above.

Organisations for Parents Under Stress (OPUS—a federation of local groups which run anonymous telephone helplines). For details of local groups telephone Hornchurch (49) 51538; or write to 29 Newmarket Way, Hornchurch, Essex.

Stillbirth and Neonatal Death Society (parent-to-parent support), Argyle House, 29–31 Euston Road, London NW1 2SD [this address is shared with NAWCH (above)] (01–794–4601).

Twins Clubs Association (encouragement and support to parents of twins, triplets, or more). An s.a.e. sent to the Distribution Secretary at 10 Tolpuddle Way, Yateley, Camberley, Surrey, would enable you to make contact with your nearest local branch.

There are several thousand self-help groups and associations, national, or locally based; and new ones, for instance to support parents of a baby born with a little-known medical condition, come into existence every day. For information contact the Postnatal Committee at the NCT's London address and they will do their best to help.

Further reading

(In each case the date given is that of first publication)

ANTENATAL

Close, Sylvia, *The Know-how of Pregnancy and Labour* (Wright, 1975)

—*Birth Report* (National Foundation for Educational Research, 1979)

—*Sex during Pregnancy and after Childbirth* (Thorsons, 1984)

Dick-Read, Grantley, *Childbirth without Fear* (Piper, 1969)

Inch, Sally, *Birthrights* (Hutchinson, 1982)

Karmel, Marjorie, *Babies without Tears* (Secker & Warburg, 1971)

Kitzinger, Sheila, *Birth at Home* (Oxford University Press, 1979)

—*The Experience of Childbirth* (2nd edn., Gollancz, 1972)

—*Giving Birth: Parents' Emotions in Childbirth* (Gollancz/Sphere, 1971)

Leboyer, Frederick, *Birth without Violence* (Wildwood House/Fontana, 1975)

Lewis, Catherine, *Good Food Before Birth* (Unwin Paperbacks, 1984)

Llewellyn-Jones, Derek: *Everywoman: A Gynaecological Guide for Life* (2nd edn., Faber, 1978)

Lux Flanagan, Geraldine, *The First Nine Months of Life* (Heinemann Medical, 1963)

Madders, Jane, *Stress and Relaxation* (Martin Dunitz, 1979)

Macfarlane, Aidan, *The Psychology of Childbirth* (Fontana/Open Books, 1977)

Milinaire, Caterine, *Birth* (Omnibus, 1976)

Nilsson, Lennart, *et al.*, *The Everyday Miracle* (Faber/Penguin, 1977)

Noble, Elizabeth, *Essential Exercises for the Childbearing Year* (2nd edn., John Murray, 1980)

Odent, Michel, *Birth Reborn* (Souvenir Press, 1984)

Pickard, Barbara, *Food, Health and having a Baby* (Sheldon, 1984)

Verny, Thomas, *The Secret Life of the Unborn Child* (Sphere, 1982)

Wright, Erna, *The New Childbirth* (Tandem, 1969)

POSTNATAL and FEEDING

Bell, Joyce and Michael, *The Baby in the Bubble* (Oxford School Publications, 1980; available from Bridge House, Witney, Oxon. OX8 6HY)

Clapham NCT Working Mothers Group, *The Working Mother's Handbook* (available from 167 Fentiman Road, London SW8 1JY)

Close, Sylvia, *The Know-how of Breast-Feeding* (Wright, 1972)

—*The Know-how of Infant Care* (Wright, 1972)

—*The Know-how of Infant Feeding* (Wright, 1973)

—*The Toddler and the New Baby* (Routledge, 1980)

Douglas, Jo, and Richman, Naomi, *My Child Won't Sleep* (Penguin, 1984)

Eiger, Marvin S., and Olds, Sally W., *The Complete Book of Breast-Feeding* (Bantam, 1974)

Kitzinger, Sheila, *The Experience of Breastfeeding* (Penguin Books, 1979)

La Leche League International, *The Womanly Art of Breast-Feeding* (Souvenir Press/Tandem, 1970)

Leboyer, Frederick, *Loving Hands* (Collins, 1977)

Lewis, Catherine (ed.), *Growing up with Good Food* (Unwin Paperbacks in association with The National Childbirth Trust, 1982)

Mansfield, Peter, *Common Sense About Health* (Templegarth Trust, 1982)

Messenger, Maire, *The Breastfeeding Book* (Century, 1982)

Montgomery, Eileen, *Regaining Bladder Control* (Wright, 1983)

McKenna, Polden, and Williams, *You—after Childbirth* (Churchill Livingstone, 1980)

Stanway, Penny and Andrew, *Breast is Best* (Pan, 1978)

Index